Breakfasts for a Fresh Start

Light and Nourishing Lunches

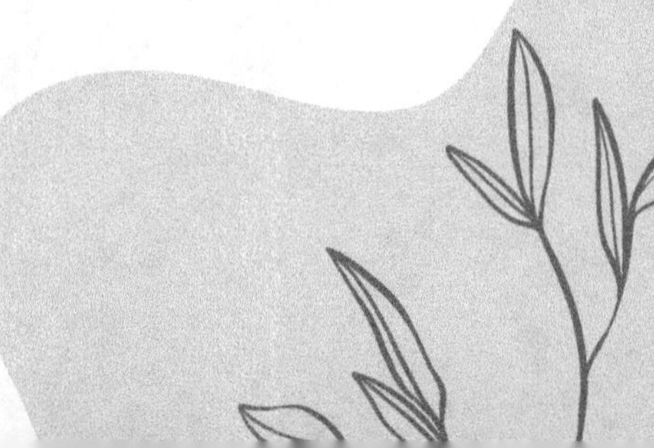

Balanced Dinners

Sides and Snacks

Sweet and Healthy Desserts

Understanding Menopause

Menopause is a natural biological process that marks the end of a woman's menstrual cycles. It typically occurs in women in their late 40s to early 50s, although it can happen earlier or later. Menopause is officially diagnosed after a woman has gone 12 months without a menstrual period. This transition period leading up to menopause, known as perimenopause, can bring a variety of physical and emotional changes.

Symptoms of Menopause

During menopause, women may experience a range of symptoms including hot flashes, night sweats, mood swings, weight gain, and changes in libido. These symptoms are primarily caused by fluctuating hormone levels, particularly a decrease in estrogen and progesterone.

Health Implications

The decline in estrogen levels can also affect long-term health. Postmenopausal women are at an increased risk for osteoporosis, heart disease, and other health conditions. Therefore, maintaining a healthy diet and lifestyle is crucial during this stage of life.

Benefits of a Menopause Diet

Adopting a menopause-friendly diet can help manage symptoms and reduce the risk of chronic diseases. A balanced diet rich in whole foods, lean proteins, healthy fats, and plenty of fruits and vegetables can provide essential nutrients that support overall health and well-being during menopause.

Key Nutrients

Certain nutrients are particularly beneficial during menopause:

- Calcium and Vitamin D: Essential for bone health to prevent osteoporosis.

- Phytoestrogens: Found in soy products, flaxseeds, and legumes, these can mimic estrogen and help balance hormone levels.

- Omega-3 Fatty Acids: Found in fish, walnuts, and flaxseeds, these can reduce inflammation and support heart health.

- Fiber: Helps with digestion and can aid in weight management.

- B Vitamins: Important for energy production and can help with mood regulation.

How to Use This Cookbook

This cookbook is designed to provide you with delicious and nutritious recipes that cater specifically to the needs of women going through menopause. Each recipe is carefully crafted to include ingredients that support hormone balance, bone health, and overall well-being.

Recipe Categories

The recipes are divided into several categories to help you find what you need easily:

- Breakfasts for a Fresh Start: Energizing and nutrient-dense options to start your day right.

- Light and Nourishing Lunches: Wholesome meals that keep you satisfied without feeling heavy.

- Balanced Dinners: Protein-rich and vegetable-packed dishes for your evening meal.

- Sides and Snacks: Healthy options to complement your meals or to enjoy between them.

- Comforting Soups and Stews: Warm and hearty recipes perfect for any time of the year.

- Sweet and Healthy Desserts: Guilt-free treats that satisfy your sweet tooth.

- Beverages and Smoothies: Hydrating and nutritious drinks to keep you refreshed.

Tips for Success

- Plan Ahead: Meal planning can help you stay on track with your dietary goals and make grocery shopping more efficient.

- Stay Hydrated: Drink plenty of water throughout the day to support overall health and well-being.

- Listen to Your Body: Pay attention to how different foods affect your symptoms and adjust your diet accordingly.

- Stay Active: Combine a healthy diet with regular physical activity to maintain strength, flexibility, and overall fitness.

Embarking on a menopause diet is a journey towards better health and well-being. This cookbook aims to empower you with the knowledge and tools to make informed dietary choices that can help manage menopause symptoms and improve your quality of life. Enjoy the delicious recipes and embrace the positive changes that come with nourishing your body during this significant life transition.

Welcome to "The New Menopause Diet Cookbook." Let's get started on this healthy and flavorful journey together!

1. Greek Yogurt with Berries and Flaxseeds

Ingredients:

- 1 cup plain Greek yogurt
- 1/2 cup mixed berries
 (such as blueberries, raspberries, blackberries)
- 1 tablespoon ground flaxseeds

Instructions:

1. In a medium bowl, scoop the Greek yogurt.

2. Top the yogurt with the mixed berries.

3. Sprinkle the ground flaxseeds over the top.

4. Stir the ingredients together gently until well combined.

5. Serve immediately or refrigerate until ready to enjoy.

This quick and easy recipe makes for a nutritious and delicious breakfast or snack. The Greek yogurt provides protein, the berries add natural sweetness and antioxidants, and the flaxseeds contribute fiber, omega-3 fatty acids, and a nutty flavor. Adjust the amounts of each ingredient to your personal taste preferences.

PreparationTime: 5 minutes
Cook Time: 0 minutes
Total Time: 5 minutes
Serves: 1

2. Overnight Oats with Chia Seeds and Fresh Fruit

Ingredients:

- 1/2 cup old-fashioned rolled oats
- 1 tablespoon chia seeds
- 1/2 cup unsweetened almond milk
 (or milk of your choice)
- 1 tablespoon maple syrup (optional)
- 1/2 cup mixed fresh fruit
 (such as berries, sliced banana, diced apple)

PreparationTime: 5 minutes
Refrigeration Time: 8 hours or overnight
Total Time: 8 hours 5 minutes
Serves: 1

Instructions:

1. In a medium bowl or mason jar, combine the rolled oats and chia seeds.

2. Pour in the almond milk and stir to combine. If using, drizzle in the maple syrup and stir again.

3. Cover the bowl or seal the mason jar and refrigerate for at least 8 hours, or overnight.

4. In the morning, remove the overnight oats from the refrigerator. Top with the mixed fresh fruit.

5. Stir everything together and enjoy cold.

The oats will have absorbed the milk, creating a creamy, pudding-like texture. The chia seeds will have expanded, adding fiber and nutrients. The fresh fruit provides natural sweetness, vitamins, and antioxidants. This make-ahead breakfast is nutritious, delicious, and perfect for busy mornings.

3. Scrambled Eggs with Spinach and Tomatoes

Ingredients:

- 4 large eggs
- 2 tablespoons milk
- 1/4 teaspoon salt
- 1/8 teaspoon black pepper
- 1 tablespoon olive oil
- 1 cup fresh spinach, chopped
- 1 cup cherry tomatoes, halved

PreparationTime: 5 minutes
Cook Time: 10 minutes
Total Time: 15 minutes
Serves: 2

Instructions:

1. In a medium bowl, whisk together the eggs, milk, salt, and pepper until well combined.

2. Heat the olive oil in a nonstick skillet over medium heat.

3. Add the chopped spinach to the skillet and cook for 2-3 minutes, stirring occasionally, until the spinach is wilted.

4. Pour the egg mixture into the skillet with the spinach. Use a spatula to gently push and fold the eggs as they cook, creating soft, fluffy curds.

5. Once the eggs are nearly cooked through, add the halved cherry tomatoes to the skillet. Cook for an additional 1-2 minutes, continuing to fold the eggs, until they are fully cooked.

6. Remove the skillet from heat and serve the scrambled eggs with spinach and tomatoes immediately.

This nutritious scramble is packed with protein from the eggs, vitamins and minerals from the spinach, and juicy sweetness from the tomatoes. It makes a delicious and satisfying breakfast or brunch.

4. Avocado Toast with Poached Eggs

Ingredients:

- 2 large eggs
- 2 slices whole grain bread, toasted
- 1 ripe avocado, mashed
- 1 tablespoon olive oil
- 1 tablespoon white vinegar
- Salt and pepper to taste
- Red pepper flakes (optional)

PreparationTime: 10 minutes
Cook Time: 5 minutes
Total Time: 15 minutes
Serves: 2

Instructions:

1. Bring a medium saucepan of water to a gentle simmer over medium heat. Add the white vinegar.

2. Crack the eggs one at a time into a small bowl or ramekin, then gently slide them into the simmering water. Poach the eggs for 3-5 minutes, until the whites are set but the yolks are still runny.

3. Using a slotted spoon, remove the poached eggs from the water and set aside.

4. Toast the bread slices until golden brown.

5. Spread the mashed avocado evenly over the toasted bread slices.

6. Top each avocado toast with a poached egg.

7. Drizzle the avocado toasts with olive oil and season with salt and pepper to taste.

8. Sprinkle with red pepper flakes, if desired.

9. Serve the avocado toast with poached eggs immediately.

This nutrient-dense breakfast combines the healthy fats from avocado, the protein from eggs, and the fiber from whole grain bread. It's a delicious and satisfying way to start your day.

5. Smoothie with Spinach, Banana, and Almond Milk

Ingredients:

- 1 cup unsweetened almond milk
- 1 cup fresh spinach leaves
- 1 ripe banana, frozen
- 1 tablespoon ground flaxseeds
- 1 teaspoon honey (optional)

PreparationTime: 5 minutes
Total Time: 5 minutes
Serves: 1

Instructions:

1. In a high-powered blender, combine the almond milk, spinach, frozen banana, and ground flaxseeds.

2. Blend on high speed until the mixture is smooth and creamy, about 1-2 minutes.

3. Taste the smoothie and add honey if desired, blending again briefly to incorporate.

4. Pour the smoothie into a glass and enjoy immediately.

This smoothie is an excellent choice for a menopause diet for a few reasons:

- Spinach is rich in vitamins and minerals like iron, calcium, and magnesium, which can help support bone health during menopause.

- Bananas are a good source of potassium, which can help regulate blood pressure and reduce the risk of heart disease.

- Almond milk is low in calories and fat, but high in calcium, vitamin E, and other nutrients that are beneficial during menopause.

- Flaxseeds provide fiber, omega-3 fatty acids, and phytoestrogens, which may help alleviate some menopausal symptoms.

The honey is optional, but can add a touch of natural sweetness if desired. This smoothie makes a nutritious and delicious breakfast or snack.

6. Cottage Cheese with Pineapple and Chia Seeds

Ingredients:

- 1 cup low-fat cottage cheese
- 1/2 cup fresh pineapple, diced
- 1 tablespoon chia seeds
- 1 teaspoon honey (optional)

PreparationTime: 5 minutes
Total Time: 5 minutes
Serves: 1

Instructions:

1. In a medium bowl, combine the cottage cheese, diced pineapple, and chia seeds.

2. Stir the ingredients together until well mixed.

3. If desired, drizzle the honey over the top and stir again gently to incorporate.

4. Serve immediately or refrigerate until ready to enjoy.

This simple, nutrient-dense snack or light meal is an excellent choice for a menopause diet for several reasons:

- Cottage cheese is a great source of protein, which can help maintain muscle mass and bone health during menopause.
- Pineapple is rich in vitamin C, an antioxidant that may help reduce the risk of certain health issues associated with menopause.
- Chia seeds are high in fiber, omega-3 fatty acids, and phytoestrogens, which may help alleviate menopausal symptoms.
- The honey (if used) provides a touch of natural sweetness without adding too many calories.

The combination of protein, fiber, and healthy fats in this dish can help keep you feeling full and satisfied, while also providing important nutrients that support overall health during menopause. Adjust the amounts of each ingredient to your personal taste preferences.

7. Protein Pancakes with Blueberries

Ingredients:

- 1/2 cup rolled oats
- 2 large eggs
- 1/4 cup unsweetened almond milk
- 1 tablespoon ground flaxseed
- 1 teaspoon baking powder
- 1/4 teaspoon ground cinnamon
- 1/4 teaspoon vanilla extract
- 1 cup fresh or frozen blueberries

PreparationTime: 10 minutes
Cook Time: 10 minutes
Total Time: 20 minutes
Serves: 2 (2-3 pancakes per serving)

Instructions:

1. In a blender, combine the rolled oats, eggs, almond milk, flaxseed, baking powder, cinnamon, and vanilla extract. Blend until the batter is smooth and well combined.

2. Heat a nonstick skillet or griddle over medium heat. Lightly grease the surface with a small amount of cooking spray or oil.

3. Scoop the batter onto the hot surface, using about 1/4 cup of batter per pancake. Gently press a few blueberries into the top of each pancake.

4. Cook the pancakes for 2-3 minutes per side, or until golden brown and cooked through.

5. Serve the protein pancakes warm, with additional blueberries on top if desired.

These protein-packed pancakes are an excellent choice for a menopause diet for several reasons:

- Oats and eggs provide high-quality protein to help maintain muscle mass.
- Blueberries are rich in antioxidants and may help reduce inflammation.
- Flaxseed is a good source of fiber, omega-3 fatty acids, and phytoestrogens.
- Cinnamon may help regulate blood sugar levels.

This balanced breakfast can help provide sustained energy and support overall health during menopause. Adjust the amount of batter or number of pancakes per serving to suit your appetite.

8. Quinoa Breakfast Bowl with Almonds and Honey

Ingredients:

- 1/2 cup cooked quinoa, cooled
- 1/2 cup unsweetened almond milk
- 2 tablespoons sliced almonds
- 1 tablespoon honey
- 1/4 teaspoon ground cinnamon
- Pinch of salt

PreparationTime: 5 minutes
Cook Time: 15 minutes
Total Time: 20 minutes
Serves: 1

Instructions:

1. In a medium bowl, combine the cooked quinoa, almond milk, sliced almonds, honey, cinnamon, and a pinch of salt. Stir well to mix.

2. Microwave the quinoa mixture for 1-2 minutes, or until heated through.

3. Carefully remove the bowl from the microwave and give it another stir.

4. Serve the quinoa breakfast bowl warm, with additional honey drizzled on top if desired.

This quinoa breakfast bowl is a nutritious and satisfying way to start your day. Here's why it's a great choice:

- Quinoa is a complete protein, providing all the essential amino acids. It's also high in fiber, vitamins, and minerals.
- Almonds are a good source of healthy fats, protein, and antioxidants.
- Honey provides natural sweetness and contains antioxidants.
- Cinnamon may help regulate blood sugar levels.
- Almond milk is low in calories but high in calcium and other nutrients.

The combination of complex carbs, protein, healthy fats, and fiber in this dish can help keep you feeling full and energized throughout the morning. Adjust the amounts of each ingredient to your personal taste preferences.

9. Chia Pudding with Fresh Berries

Ingredients:

- 2 tablespoons chia seeds
- 1/2 cup unsweetened almond milk
- 1 tablespoon maple syrup (optional)
- 1/2 cup mixed fresh berries
 (such as raspberries, blueberries, strawberries)

PreparationTime: 5 minutes
Refrigeration Time: 4 hours or overnight
Total Time: 4 hours 5 minutes
Serves: 1

Instructions:

1. In a small bowl or mason jar, combine the chia seeds and almond milk. Stir well.

2. If using, drizzle in the maple syrup and stir again to incorporate.

3. Cover the bowl or seal the mason jar and refrigerate for at least 4 hours, or overnight.

4. When ready to serve, remove the chia pudding from the refrigerator. The chia seeds will have expanded, creating a thick, pudding-like consistency.

5. Top the chia pudding with the mixed fresh berries.

6. Serve chilled.

This chia pudding is an excellent choice for a menopause diet for several reasons:

- Chia seeds are high in fiber, protein, omega-3 fatty acids, and phytoestrogens, which may help alleviate menopausal symptoms.
- Berries are rich in antioxidants, vitamins, and minerals that can support overall health during menopause.
- Almond milk is low in calories and fat but high in calcium, vitamin E, and other nutrients.
- The maple syrup (if used) provides a touch of natural sweetness without adding too many calories.

The make-ahead nature of this recipe also makes it a convenient and nutritious breakfast or snack option. Adjust the amount of maple syrup to your personal taste preferences.

10. Almond Butter and Banana on Whole Grain Toast

Ingredients:

- 2 slices whole grain bread, toasted
- 2 tablespoons creamy almond butter
- 1 ripe banana, sliced

PreparationTime: 5 minutes
Total Time: 5 minutes
Serves: 1

Instructions:

1. Toast the whole grain bread slices until golden brown.

2. Spread the almond butter evenly over the toasted bread slices.

3. Arrange the sliced banana on top of the almond butter.

4. Serve the almond butter and banana toast immediately.

This simple, nutrient-dense snack or light meal is an excellent choice for a menopause diet for several reasons:

- Whole grain bread provides complex carbohydrates, fiber, and B vitamins, which can help support energy levels and overall health.
- Almond butter is a good source of protein, healthy fats, and minerals like magnesium and calcium, which are important during menopause.
- Bananas are rich in potassium, which can help regulate blood pressure and reduce the risk of heart disease.

The combination of complex carbs, protein, and healthy fats in this dish can help keep you feeling full and satisfied, while also providing important nutrients that support overall health during menopause. You can adjust the amounts of almond butter and banana to your personal taste preferences.

This quick and easy snack or breakfast is a great way to start your day or refuel during the afternoon. It's a nutritious and delicious option for a menopause diet.

11. Veggie Omelette with Mushrooms and Peppers

Ingredients:

- 2 large eggs
- 1 tablespoon milk or unsweetened almond milk
- 1/4 teaspoon salt
- 1/8 teaspoon black pepper
- 1 teaspoon olive oil
- 1/4 cup sliced mushrooms
- 1/4 cup diced bell pepper (any color)
- 1 tablespoon shredded cheddar cheese (optional)

PreparationTime: 10 minutes
Cook Time: 10 minutes
Total Time: 20 minutes
Serves: 1

Instructions:

1. In a small bowl, whisk together the eggs, milk, salt, and pepper until well combined.

2. Heat the olive oil in a nonstick skillet over medium heat.

3. Add the sliced mushrooms and diced bell pepper to the skillet. Sauté for 2-3 minutes, until the vegetables are tender.

4. Pour the egg mixture into the skillet, tilting the pan to allow the uncooked egg to flow to the edges.

5. As the eggs start to set, use a spatula to gently push the cooked egg towards the center, tilting the pan to allow the uncooked egg to flow to the edges.

6. Once the eggs are mostly set but still slightly runny on top, sprinkle the shredded cheddar cheese (if using) over the top. Fold the omelette in half and slide it onto a plate. Serve immediately.

This veggie-packed omelette is an excellent choice for a menopause diet for several reasons:

- Eggs are a great source of protein, which can help maintain muscle mass and bone health.
- Mushrooms and bell peppers are rich in antioxidants, vitamins, and minerals that can support overall health. The cheese (if used) provides additional protein and calcium, which is important during menopause.

This balanced meal offers a combination of protein, fiber, and nutrients that can help keep you feeling full and energized throughout the day. Adjust the amount of vegetables or cheese to your personal taste preferences.

12. Whole Grain Waffles with Greek Yogurt and Strawberries

Ingredients:

- 1 cup whole wheat flour
- 1 teaspoon baking powder
- 1/4 teaspoon salt
- 1 egg
- 1 cup unsweetened almond milk
- 1 tablespoon honey
- 1 cup plain Greek yogurt
- 1 cup fresh strawberries, sliced

Breakfasts for a Fresh Start

PreparationTime: 10 minutes
Cook Time: 10 minutes
Total Time: 20 minutes
Serves: 2 (2 waffles per serving)

Instructions:

1. Preheat a waffle iron according to the manufacturer's instructions.

2. In a medium bowl, whisk together the whole wheat flour, baking powder, and salt.

3. In a separate bowl, beat the egg. Then stir in the almond milk and honey until well combined.

4. Pour the wet ingredients into the dry ingredients and stir just until combined (do not overmix).

5. Lightly grease the preheated waffle iron. Scoop the batter onto the iron, using about 1/2 cup of batter per waffle.

6. Cook the waffles for 4-5 minutes, or until golden brown and crispy.

7. Remove the waffles from the iron and place them on plates. Top each waffle with a dollop of Greek yogurt and sliced fresh strawberries. Serve the whole grain waffles with Greek yogurt and strawberries immediately.

This nutrient-dense breakfast is an excellent choice for a menopause diet for several reasons:

- Whole wheat flour provides complex carbohydrates, fiber, and B vitamins.
- Greek yogurt is high in protein, which can help maintain muscle mass.
- Strawberries are rich in antioxidants, vitamins, and fiber.
- Honey provides natural sweetness without added refined sugars.

The combination of complex carbs, protein, and healthy fats in this dish can help keep you feeling full and satisfied, while also providing important nutrients that support overall health during menopause. Adjust the amounts of toppings to your personal taste preferences.

13. Apple Cinnamon Overnight Oats

Ingredients:

- 1/2 cup old-fashioned rolled oats
- 1/2 cup unsweetened almond milk
- 1 tablespoon chia seeds
- 1 teaspoon ground cinnamon
- 1 tablespoon maple syrup (optional)
- 1/2 cup diced apple

Breakfasts for a Fresh Start

PreparationTime: 5 minutes
Refrigeration Time: 8 hours or overnight
Total Time: 8 hours 5 minutes
Serves: 1

Instructions:

1. In a medium bowl or mason jar, combine the rolled oats, almond milk, chia seeds, and cinnamon. Stir to mix well.

2. If using, drizzle the maple syrup over the oat mixture and stir again to incorporate.

3. Fold in the diced apple.

4. Cover the bowl or seal the mason jar and refrigerate for at least 8 hours, or overnight.

5. In the morning, remove the apple cinnamon overnight oats from the refrigerator.

6. Stir the oats briefly before serving. The oats will have absorbed the liquid, creating a creamy, pudding-like texture.

This apple cinnamon overnight oats recipe is an excellent choice for a menopause diet for several reasons:

- Oats are a good source of complex carbohydrates, fiber, and beta-glucan, which can help support heart health.
- Chia seeds are high in fiber, protein, and omega-3 fatty acids, which may help alleviate menopausal symptoms.
- Cinnamon may help regulate blood sugar levels and reduce inflammation.
- Apples are rich in antioxidants, vitamins, and fiber, which can support overall health during menopause.
- The maple syrup (if used) provides a touch of natural sweetness without added refined sugars.

The make-ahead nature of this recipe also makes it a convenient and nutritious breakfast option. Adjust the amount of maple syrup to your personal taste preferences.

14. Pumpkin Spice Smoothie

Ingredients:

- 1/2 cup unsweetened almond milk
- 1/2 cup plain Greek yogurt
- 1/2 cup canned pumpkin puree
- 1 tablespoon ground flaxseed
- 1 teaspoon honey (optional)
- 1/2 teaspoon pumpkin pie spice
- 1/4 teaspoon ground cinnamon

PreparationTime: 5 minutes
Total Time: 5 minutes
Serves: 1

Instructions:

1. In a high-powered blender, combine the almond milk, Greek yogurt, pumpkin puree, ground flaxseed, honey (if using), pumpkin pie spice, and cinnamon.

2. Blend on high speed until the mixture is smooth and creamy, about 1-2 minutes.

3. Pour the pumpkin spice smoothie into a glass and serve immediately.

This pumpkin spice smoothie is an excellent choice for a menopause diet for several reasons:

- Pumpkin is rich in vitamins A and C, as well as fiber, which can help support overall health during menopause.
- Greek yogurt provides protein to help maintain muscle mass.
- Flaxseed is a good source of fiber, omega-3 fatty acids, and phytoestrogens, which may help alleviate menopausal symptoms.
- Cinnamon may help regulate blood sugar levels and reduce inflammation.
- The honey (if used) adds a touch of natural sweetness without too many calories.

The combination of nutrients in this smoothie can help keep you feeling full and energized throughout the day. Adjust the amount of honey to your personal taste preferences. You can also add a handful of spinach or kale for an extra nutrient boost.

This pumpkin spice smoothie is a delicious and nutritious option for a menopause diet.

15. Smoked Salmon and Avocado on Rye Bread

Ingredients:

- 2 slices rye bread, toasted
- 2 ounces smoked salmon
- 1/2 ripe avocado, sliced
- 1 tablespoon fresh dill, chopped
- 1 tablespoon lemon juice
- Salt and pepper to taste

PreparationTime: 5 minutes
Total Time: 5 minutes
Serves: 1

Instructions:

1. Toast the rye bread slices until golden brown.

2. Arrange the smoked salmon on one slice of toast.

3. Top the salmon with the sliced avocado.

4. Sprinkle the chopped fresh dill over the avocado.

5. Drizzle the lemon juice over the top.

6. Season with a pinch of salt and pepper. Top with the remaining slice of toast. Serve the smoked salmon and avocado open-faced sandwich immediately.

This nutrient-dense open-faced sandwich is an excellent choice for a menopause diet for several reasons:

- Rye bread is a whole grain that provides complex carbohydrates, fiber, and B vitamins.
- Smoked salmon is a great source of protein and omega-3 fatty acids, which can help support heart and brain health.
- Avocado is rich in healthy monounsaturated fats, as well as vitamins, minerals, and antioxidants.
- Dill and lemon juice add flavor and provide additional antioxidant benefits.

The combination of protein, healthy fats, and complex carbs in this dish can help keep you feeling full and satisfied, while also providing important nutrients that support overall health during menopause. Adjust the amounts of each ingredient to your personal taste preferences.

This open-faced sandwich makes for a quick and nutritious breakfast, lunch, or snack option for a menopause diet.

16. Breakfast Burrito with Eggs, Black Beans, and Salsa

Ingredients:

- 1 whole wheat tortilla
- 2 large eggs, scrambled
- 1/2 cup canned black beans, rinsed and heated
- 2 tablespoons salsa
- 1 tablespoon shredded cheddar cheese (optional)
- 1 tablespoon diced avocado (optional)

PreparationTime: 10 minutes
Cook Time: 10 minutes
Total Time: 20 minutes
Serves: 1

Instructions:

1. In a nonstick skillet, scramble the eggs over medium heat until cooked through, about 2-3 minutes.

2. Warm the whole wheat tortilla according to package instructions.

3. Place the scrambled eggs in the center of the tortilla.

4. Top the eggs with the heated black beans, salsa, shredded cheddar cheese (if using), and diced avocado (if using).

5. Fold the bottom of the tortilla up, then fold in the sides and continue rolling to create a burrito shape.

6. Serve the breakfast burrito immediately.

This breakfast burrito is an excellent choice for a menopause diet for several reasons:

- Whole wheat tortillas provide complex carbohydrates, fiber, and B vitamins.
- Eggs are a great source of protein, which can help maintain muscle mass and bone health.
- Black beans are high in fiber, protein, and minerals like iron and magnesium.
- Salsa adds flavor and provides antioxidants from the tomatoes and other vegetables.
- Avocado and cheddar cheese (if used) contribute healthy fats and additional nutrients.

The combination of protein, fiber, and complex carbs in this dish can help keep you feeling full and energized throughout the morning. Adjust the amounts of the fillings to your personal taste preferences.

This breakfast burrito is a nutritious and portable option for a menopause diet.

17. Whole Grain Cereal with Almond Milk and Fresh Fruit

Ingredients:

- 1 cup unsweetened almond milk
- 3/4 cup whole grain cereal
(such as oats, quinoa, or millet)
- 1/2 cup mixed fresh fruit
(such as berries, sliced banana, diced apple)
- 1 tablespoon ground flaxseed (optional)
- 1 teaspoon honey (optional)

PreparationTime: 5 minutes
Total Time: 5 minutes
Serves: 1

Instructions:

1. In a bowl, pour the unsweetened almond milk over the whole grain cereal.

2. Top the cereal with the mixed fresh fruit.

3. If using, sprinkle the ground flaxseed over the top.

4. Drizzle the honey over the fruit and cereal, if desired.

5. Stir everything together gently until well combined. Serve the whole grain cereal with almond milk and fresh fruit immediately.

This simple, nutrient-dense breakfast is an excellent choice for a menopause diet for several reasons:

- Whole grain cereals like oats, quinoa, and millet provide complex carbohydrates, fiber, and important vitamins and minerals.
- Almond milk is low in calories and fat but high in calcium, vitamin E, and other nutrients.
- Fresh fruit adds natural sweetness, vitamins, and antioxidants.
- Flaxseed is a good source of fiber, omega-3 fatty acids, and phytoestrogens, which may help alleviate menopausal symptoms.
- Honey (if used) provides a touch of natural sweetness without added refined sugars.

The combination of complex carbs, protein, fiber, and healthy fats in this dish can help keep you feeling full and satisfied, while also providing important nutrients that support overall health during menopause. Adjust the amounts of each ingredient to your personal taste preferences.

This whole grain cereal with almond milk and fresh fruit makes for a quick, easy, and nutritious breakfast option for a menopause diet.

18. Baked Egg Cups with Veggies

Ingredients:

- 8 large eggs
- 1/4 cup unsweetened almond milk
- 1/4 teaspoon salt
- 1/8 teaspoon black pepper
- 1 cup diced bell peppers
- 1/2 cup diced mushrooms
- 1/2 cup chopped spinach
- 2 tablespoons shredded cheddar cheese (optional)

PreparationTime: 10 minutes
Cook Time: 20 minutes
Total Time: 30 minutes
Serves: 4 (2 egg cups per serving)

Instructions:

1. Preheat the oven to 375°F. Grease a 12-cup muffin tin with nonstick cooking spray.

2. In a medium bowl, whisk together the eggs, almond milk, salt, and pepper until well combined.

3. Divide the diced bell peppers, mushrooms, and chopped spinach evenly among the prepared muffin cups.

4. Carefully pour the egg mixture over the vegetables, filling each cup about 3/4 full.

5. If using, sprinkle the shredded cheddar cheese on top of the egg cups.

6. Bake for 18-20 minutes, or until the eggs are set and the edges are lightly golden.

7. Remove the baked egg cups from the oven and let them cool in the muffin tin for 5 minutes.

8. Use a fork or spoon to gently remove the egg cups from the tin.

9. Serve the baked egg cups warm.

The combination of protein, fiber, and nutrients in these baked egg cups can help keep you feeling full and energized throughout the morning. Adjust the types and amounts of vegetables to your personal taste preferences.

This make-ahead breakfast is a convenient and nutritious option for a menopause diet.

19. Green Smoothie Bowl with Toppings

Ingredients:

Smoothie:
- 1 cup unsweetened almond milk
- 1 cup packed baby spinach
- 1 frozen banana
- 1 tablespoon ground flaxseed
- 1 teaspoon honey (optional)

PreparationTime: 10 minutes
Total Time: 10 minutes
Serves: 1

Toppings:
- 1/4 cup fresh berries (such as blueberries, raspberries, or sliced strawberries)
- 2 tablespoons chopped walnuts
- 1 tablespoon unsweetened shredded coconut
- 1 teaspoon chia seeds

Instructions:

1. In a high-powered blender, combine the almond milk, spinach, frozen banana, ground flaxseed, and honey (if using). Blend on high speed until smooth and creamy.

2. Pour the green smoothie into a bowl.

3. Top the smoothie with the fresh berries, chopped walnuts, shredded coconut, and chia seeds. Serve the green smoothie bowl immediately.

This nutrient-dense smoothie bowl is an excellent choice for a menopause diet for several reasons:

- Spinach is packed with vitamins, minerals, and antioxidants that can support overall health.
- Bananas provide potassium, which can help regulate blood pressure.
- Flaxseed is a good source of fiber, omega-3 fatty acids, and phytoestrogens that may help alleviate menopausal symptoms.
- Berries are rich in antioxidants and can help reduce inflammation.
- Walnuts contain healthy fats, protein, and magnesium, which is important during menopause.
- Chia seeds and coconut provide additional fiber, protein, and healthy fats.

This green smoothie bowl makes for a nutritious and satisfying breakfast or snack.

20. Steel-Cut Oats with Walnuts and Maple Syrup

Ingredients:

- 1 cup unsweetened almond milk
- 1 cup water
- 1/2 cup steel-cut oats
- 1/4 teaspoon ground cinnamon
- 1 tablespoon chopped walnuts
- 1 tablespoon pure maple syrup (optional)

PreparationTime: 5 minutes
Cook Time: 20 minutes
Total Time: 25 minutes
Serves: 2

Instructions:

1. In a medium saucepan, bring the almond milk and water to a boil over high heat.

2. Once boiling, stir in the steel-cut oats and cinnamon. Reduce the heat to medium-low and let the oats simmer, stirring occasionally, for 18-20 minutes, until thickened to your desired consistency.

3. Remove the saucepan from the heat. Stir in the chopped walnuts.

4. If using, drizzle the maple syrup over the top of the oatmeal.

5. Serve the steel-cut oats with walnuts and maple syrup warm.

This hearty oatmeal dish is an excellent choice for a menopause diet for several reasons:

- Steel-cut oats are a whole grain that provide complex carbohydrates, fiber, and B vitamins.
- Walnuts are a good source of protein, healthy fats, and magnesium, which is important during menopause.
- Cinnamon may help regulate blood sugar levels and reduce inflammation.
- Maple syrup (if used) provides a touch of natural sweetness without added refined sugars.
- Almond milk is low in calories and fat but high in calcium and other nutrients.

The combination of complex carbs, protein, fiber, and healthy fats in this dish can help keep you feeling full and satisfied, while also providing important nutrients that support overall health during menopause. Adjust the amount of maple syrup to your personal taste preferences.

21. Quinoa Salad with Chickpeas, Cucumber, and Feta

Ingredients:

- 1 cup cooked quinoa, cooled
- 1 (15 oz) can chickpeas, rinsed and drained
- 1 cup diced cucumber
- 1/4 cup crumbled feta cheese
- 2 tablespoons chopped fresh parsley
- 1 tablespoon olive oil
- 1 tablespoon lemon juice
- 1/4 teaspoon salt
- 1/8 teaspoon black pepper

Instructions:

1. In a large bowl, combine the cooked quinoa, chickpeas, diced cucumber, crumbled feta, and chopped parsley.

2. Drizzle the olive oil and lemon juice over the salad. Season with salt and pepper.

3. Gently toss all the ingredients together until well mixed.

4. Serve the quinoa salad immediately or refrigerate until ready to enjoy.

This quinoa salad is an excellent choice for a menopause diet for several reasons:

- Quinoa is a complete protein, providing all the essential amino acids. It's also high in fiber, vitamins, and minerals.
- Chickpeas are a good source of plant-based protein, fiber, and complex carbohydrates.
- Cucumber provides hydration and is rich in vitamins and antioxidants.
- Feta cheese adds a boost of calcium, which is important during menopause.
- Parsley, olive oil, and lemon juice provide anti-inflammatory benefits.

The combination of complex carbs, protein, fiber, and healthy fats in this salad can help keep you feeling full and satisfied, while also providing important nutrients that support overall health during menopause. Adjust the amounts of each ingredient to your personal taste preferences.

This quinoa salad makes for a nutritious and refreshing lunch or side dish for a menopause diet.

PreparationTime: 15 minutes
Total Time: 15 minutes
Serves: 2

22. Lentil Soup with Mixed Vegetables

Ingredients:

- 1 tablespoon olive oil
- 1 onion, diced
- 3 cloves garlic, minced
- 1 cup dried brown or green lentils, rinsed
- 4 cups low-sodium vegetable broth
- 1 (14.5 oz) can diced tomatoes
- 2 cups mixed frozen vegetables (such as carrots, peas, green beans)
- 1 teaspoon dried thyme
- 1/2 teaspoon ground cumin
- 1/4 teaspoon cayenne pepper (optional)
- Salt and black pepper to taste

Light and Nourishing Lunches

PreparationTime: 15 minutes
Cook Time: 30 minutes
Total Time: 45 minutes
Serves: 4

Instructions:

1. In a large pot or Dutch oven, heat the olive oil over medium heat. Add the diced onion and sauté for 3-4 minutes until translucent.

2. Add the minced garlic and sauté for an additional minute until fragrant.

3. Stir in the rinsed lentils, vegetable broth, diced tomatoes, mixed frozen vegetables, thyme, cumin, and cayenne pepper (if using). Season with salt and black pepper to taste.

4. Bring the soup to a boil, then reduce the heat and let it simmer for 25-30 minutes, or until the lentils are tender.

5. Taste the soup and adjust seasonings as needed. Serve the lentil soup hot, garnished with additional fresh thyme or parsley if desired.

This lentil soup is an excellent choice for a menopause diet for several reasons:

- Lentils are a great source of plant-based protein, fiber, and complex carbohydrates.
- The mixed vegetables provide a variety of vitamins, minerals, and antioxidants.
- Herbs and spices like thyme, cumin, and cayenne pepper can help reduce inflammation. The soup is low in sodium and high in nutrients, making it a nutritious and satisfying meal.

The combination of protein, fiber, and complex carbs in this dish can help keep you feeling full and energized, while the nutrient-dense vegetables support overall health during menopause. Adjust the amount of cayenne pepper to your personal spice tolerance.

23. Grilled Chicken Caesar Salad

Ingredients:

- 2 boneless, skinless chicken breasts
- 1 tablespoon olive oil
- 1/4 teaspoon salt
- 1/8 teaspoon black pepper
- 4 cups chopped romaine lettuce
- 2 tablespoons grated Parmesan cheese
- 2 tablespoons Caesar salad dressing (use a low-fat or yogurt-based dressing)
- 1 tablespoon toasted whole wheat croutons (optional)

PreparationTime: 15 minutes
Cook Time: 10 minutes
Total Time: 25 minutes
Serves: 2

Instructions:

1. Preheat a grill or grill pan over medium-high heat.

2. Brush the chicken breasts with the olive oil and season with salt and pepper.

3. Grill the chicken for 5-6 minutes per side, or until cooked through. Allow the chicken to rest for 5 minutes, then slice or chop it.

4. In a large bowl, combine the chopped romaine lettuce, grilled chicken, Parmesan cheese, and Caesar dressing. Toss gently to coat.

5. Top the salad with the toasted whole wheat croutons, if using. Serve the Grilled Chicken Caesar Salad immediately.

This Grilled Chicken Caesar Salad is an excellent choice for a menopause diet for several reasons:

- Chicken is a lean protein source that can help maintain muscle mass.
- Romaine lettuce is packed with vitamins, minerals, and antioxidants.
- Parmesan cheese provides calcium, which is important during menopause.
- The Caesar dressing (using a low-fat or yogurt-based version) adds flavor without too many calories or unhealthy fats.
- Whole wheat croutons provide a crunchy texture and complex carbohydrates.

The combination of protein, fiber, and nutrients in this salad can help keep you feeling full and satisfied, while also supporting overall health during menopause. Adjust the amounts of each ingredient to your personal taste preferences.

This Grilled Chicken Caesar Salad makes for a nutritious and delicious lunch or dinner option for a menopause diet.

24. Turkey and Avocado Wrap with Whole Grain Tortilla

Ingredients:

- 1 whole grain tortilla
- 2-3 ounces sliced turkey breast
- 1/2 ripe avocado, sliced
- 1 tablespoon hummus
- 1/4 cup shredded spinach or mixed greens
- 1 tablespoon crumbled feta cheese (optional)
- 1 teaspoon olive oil
- 1 teaspoon lemon juice
- Salt and pepper to taste

Light and Nourishing Lunches

PreparationTime: 10 minutes
Total Time: 10 minutes
Serves: 1

Instructions:

1. Lay the whole grain tortilla flat on a clean surface.

2. Layer the sliced turkey breast in the center of the tortilla.

3. Top the turkey with the sliced avocado, hummus, and shredded spinach or mixed greens.

4. If using, sprinkle the crumbled feta cheese over the top.

5. Drizzle the olive oil and lemon juice over the filling.

6. Season with a pinch of salt and pepper.

7. Fold the bottom of the tortilla up, then fold in the sides and continue rolling to create a wrap. Serve the turkey and avocado wrap immediately.

This wrap is an excellent choice for a menopause diet for several reasons:

- Whole grain tortillas provide complex carbohydrates, fiber, and B vitamins.
- Turkey is a lean protein source that can help maintain muscle mass.
- Avocado is rich in healthy monounsaturated fats, as well as vitamins, minerals, and antioxidants.
- Hummus adds protein and fiber from the chickpeas.
- Spinach or mixed greens are packed with vitamins, minerals, and phytonutrients.
- Feta cheese (if used) provides calcium, which is important during menopause.

This turkey and avocado wrap makes for a quick, portable, and nutritious lunch or snack option for a menopause diet.

25. Greek Salad with Grilled Chicken

Ingredients:

- 2 boneless, skinless chicken breasts
- 1 tablespoon olive oil
- 1/4 teaspoon salt
- 1/8 teaspoon black pepper
- 4 cups chopped romaine lettuce
- 1 cup cherry tomatoes, halved
- 1/2 cup diced cucumber
- 1/4 cup pitted kalamata olives, sliced
- 2 tablespoons crumbled feta cheese
- 2 tablespoons red wine vinegar
- 1 tablespoon lemon juice
- 1 teaspoon dried oregano
- 1 garlic clove, minced

PreparationTime: 15 minutes
Cook Time: 10 minutes
Total Time: 25 minutes
Serves: 2

Instructions:

1. Preheat a grill or grill pan over medium-high heat.

2. Brush the chicken breasts with the olive oil and season with salt and pepper.

3. Grill the chicken for 5-6 minutes per side, or until cooked through. Allow the chicken to rest for 5 minutes, then slice or chop it.

4. In a large bowl, combine the chopped romaine lettuce, cherry tomatoes, diced cucumber, sliced kalamata olives, and crumbled feta cheese.

5. In a small bowl, whisk together the red wine vinegar, lemon juice, dried oregano, and minced garlic.

6. Drizzle the vinaigrette over the salad and toss gently to coat.

7. Top the Greek salad with the grilled chicken. Serve the Greek Salad with Grilled Chicken immediately.

The combination of protein, fiber, healthy fats, and nutrients in this salad can help keep you feeling full and satisfied, while also supporting overall health during menopause. Adjust the amounts of the ingredients to your personal taste preferences.

This Greek Salad with Grilled Chicken makes for a nutritious and flavorful lunch or dinner option for a menopause diet.

26. Spinach and Strawberry Salad with Balsamic Vinaigrette

Ingredients:

Salad:
- 4 cups fresh spinach leaves
- 1 cup sliced fresh strawberries
- 2 tablespoons chopped walnuts
- 1 tablespoon crumbled feta cheese

PreparationTime: 10 minutes
Total Time: 10 minutes
Serves: 2

Balsamic Vinaigrette:
- 2 tablespoons balsamic vinegar
- 1 tablespoon olive oil
- 1 teaspoon Dijon mustard
- 1 teaspoon honey
- 1/4 teaspoon salt
- 1/8 teaspoon black pepper

Instructions:

1. In a large salad bowl, combine the fresh spinach leaves, sliced strawberries, chopped walnuts, and crumbled feta cheese.

2. In a small bowl, whisk together the balsamic vinegar, olive oil, Dijon mustard, honey, salt, and black pepper to make the vinaigrette.

3. Drizzle the balsamic vinaigrette over the spinach and strawberry salad, and toss gently to coat. Serve the Spinach and Strawberry Salad with Balsamic Vinaigrette immediately.

This salad is an excellent choice for a menopause diet for several reasons:

- Spinach is packed with vitamins, minerals, and antioxidants that can support overall health.
- Strawberries are rich in vitamin C, which can help reduce inflammation.
- Walnuts provide healthy fats, protein, and magnesium, which is important during menopause.
- Feta cheese adds calcium to the dish.
- The balsamic vinaigrette is made with anti-inflammatory ingredients like olive oil and Dijon mustard.

The combination of nutrient-dense greens, fresh fruit, healthy fats, and a flavorful dressing makes this salad a well-balanced and satisfying option for a menopause diet. Adjust the amounts of the ingredients to your personal taste preferences.

27. Tuna Salad with Mixed Greens

Ingredients:

- 2 (5 oz) cans tuna, drained and flaked
- 2 tablespoons mayonnaise
- 1 tablespoon Dijon mustard
- 1 tablespoon lemon juice
- 1/4 cup diced celery
- 2 tablespoons diced red onion
- Salt and pepper to taste
- 4 cups mixed greens (such as spinach, arugula, romaine)
- 1 tomato, diced
- 2 tablespoons toasted sliced almonds (optional)

Light and Nourishing Lunches

PreparationTime: 10 minutes
Cook Time: 0 minutes
Total Time: 10 minutes
Serves: 2

Instructions:

1. In a medium bowl, combine the tuna, mayonnaise, Dijon mustard, lemon juice, celery, and red onion. Season with salt and pepper to taste. Mix well.

2. Divide the mixed greens between 2 plates or bowls. Top each with half of the tuna salad mixture.

3. Sprinkle the diced tomato and toasted almonds (if using) over the top.

4. Serve immediately.

This makes a light and refreshing salad that's perfect for lunch or a light dinner. The tuna salad provides protein while the mixed greens and tomatoes add vitamins, minerals and fiber. Enjoy!

28. Hummus and Veggie Wrap

Ingredients:

- 2 whole wheat tortillas or wraps
- 1/2 cup hummus
- 1 cup mixed greens (such as spinach, arugula, kale)
- 1/2 cup sliced cucumber
- 1/2 cup sliced bell pepper
- 1/4 cup shredded carrots
- 2 tablespoons crumbled feta cheese (optional)
- 1 tablespoon lemon juice
- Salt and pepper to taste

PreparationTime: 10 minutes
Cook Time: 0 minutes
Total Time: 10 minutes
Serves: 2

Instructions:

1. Spread 1/4 cup of hummus evenly onto each tortilla or wrap, leaving a 1-inch border.

2. Layer the mixed greens, cucumber slices, bell pepper slices, and shredded carrots onto the hummus.

3. Sprinkle the feta cheese (if using) over the vegetables.

4. Drizzle 1/2 tablespoon of lemon juice over each wrap.

5. Season with salt and pepper to taste.

6. Fold the bottom of the tortilla up over the filling, then fold in the sides and continue rolling tightly into a wrap.

7. Slice the wrap in half diagonally and serve immediately.

This hummus and veggie wrap is a great option for a menopause-friendly diet. The whole wheat tortilla, hummus, and vegetables provide fiber, vitamins, and minerals to help support overall health during menopause. The lemon juice also adds a refreshing flavor and provides vitamin C. Enjoy!

29. Roasted Vegetable and Quinoa Bowl

Ingredients:

- 1 cup uncooked quinoa, rinsed
- 2 cups vegetable broth
- 1 medium zucchini, diced
- 1 medium yellow squash, diced
- 1 red bell pepper, diced
- 1 red onion, diced
- 2 tablespoons olive oil
- 1 teaspoon dried thyme
- 1 teaspoon dried oregano
- Salt and pepper to taste
- 2 cups baby spinach
- 2 tablespoons crumbled feta cheese (optional)
- 2 tablespoons toasted pumpkin seeds (optional)

Light and Nourishing Lunches

PreparationTime: 15 minutes
Cook Time: 30 minutes
Total Time: 45 minutes
Serves: 4

Instructions:

1. Preheat oven to 400°F. Line a baking sheet with parchment paper.

2. In a medium saucepan, combine the quinoa and vegetable broth. Bring to a boil, then reduce heat to low, cover and simmer for 15-20 minutes until quinoa is cooked through. Fluff with a fork.

3. In a large bowl, toss the diced zucchini, yellow squash, bell pepper and onion with the olive oil, thyme, oregano, salt and pepper.

4. Spread the vegetables in a single layer on the prepared baking sheet. Roast for 20-25 minutes, stirring halfway, until vegetables are tender and lightly browned.

5. In a large bowl, combine the cooked quinoa, roasted vegetables, baby spinach, feta cheese (if using) and pumpkin seeds (if using). Toss gently to mix.

6. Serve the roasted vegetable and quinoa bowl warm or at room temperature.

This nutrient-dense bowl is perfect for a menopause-friendly diet. The quinoa provides protein and fiber, while the roasted vegetables offer vitamins, minerals and antioxidants. The spinach, feta and pumpkin seeds add extra nutrition and texture.

30. Black Bean Soup with Cilantro

Ingredients:

- 1 tablespoon olive oil
- 1 medium onion, diced
- 3 cloves garlic, minced
- 2 teaspoons ground cumin
- 1 teaspoon dried oregano
- 1/4 teaspoon cayenne pepper (optional)
- 2 (15 oz) cans black beans, rinsed and drained
- 4 cups low-sodium vegetable or chicken broth
- 1 bay leaf
- Salt and pepper to taste
- 1/4 cup chopped fresh cilantro
- 2 tablespoons plain Greek yogurt (optional)
- Lime wedges for serving

PreparationTime: 15 minutes
Cook Time: 30 minutes
Total Time: 45 minutes
Serves: 4

Instructions:

1. In a large pot or Dutch oven, heat the olive oil over medium heat. Add the onion and sauté for 5 minutes until translucent.

2. Add the garlic, cumin, oregano and cayenne (if using). Cook for 1 minute, stirring constantly, until fragrant.

3. Add the black beans, broth and bay leaf. Bring to a boil, then reduce heat and simmer for 20-25 minutes, stirring occasionally, until slightly thickened.

4. Remove the bay leaf. Use an immersion blender to puree about half of the soup, leaving some beans whole. Alternatively, transfer 2 cups of the soup to a blender and puree, then return to the pot.

5. Season the soup with salt and pepper to taste.

6. Ladle the soup into bowls and top with chopped cilantro, a dollop of Greek yogurt (if using), and a squeeze of fresh lime juice.

This black bean soup is a great option for a menopause-friendly diet. The beans provide fiber, protein and complex carbohydrates, while the cilantro adds flavor and antioxidants. Enjoy this nourishing and comforting soup!

31. Chickpea and Avocado Salad

Ingredients:

- 1 (15 oz) can chickpeas, rinsed and drained
- 1 ripe avocado, diced
- 1/2 cup diced cucumber
- 1/4 cup diced red onion
- 2 tablespoons chopped fresh parsley
- 2 tablespoons lemon juice
- 1 tablespoon olive oil
- 1/2 teaspoon ground cumin
- 1/4 teaspoon cayenne pepper (optional)
- Salt and pepper to taste
- 2 cups mixed greens (such as spinach, arugula, kale)

PreparationTime: 15 minutes
Cook Time: 0 minutes
Total Time: 15 minutes
Serves: 4

Instructions:

1. In a large bowl, gently combine the chickpeas, avocado, cucumber, red onion and parsley.

2. In a small bowl, whisk together the lemon juice, olive oil, cumin, cayenne (if using), and a pinch of salt and pepper.

3. Pour the dressing over the chickpea and avocado mixture and toss gently to coat.

4. Divide the mixed greens between 4 plates or bowls. Top each with the chickpea and avocado salad.

5. Serve immediately.

This chickpea and avocado salad is a great option for a menopause-friendly diet. The chickpeas provide fiber, protein and complex carbohydrates, while the avocado offers healthy fats, vitamins and minerals. The mixed greens add additional nutrients and fiber. This salad is refreshing, satisfying and packed with beneficial nutrients for women during menopause.

32. Asian Chicken Salad with Sesame Dressing

Ingredients:

- 2 cups shredded cooked chicken breast
- 2 cups shredded cabbage (green or purple)
- 1 cup shredded carrots
- 1/2 cup thinly sliced red bell pepper
- 1/4 cup thinly sliced green onions
- 2 tablespoons toasted sesame seeds
- 2 tablespoons rice vinegar
- 1 tablespoon sesame oil
- 1 tablespoon low-sodium soy sauce
- 1 teaspoon honey
- 1/2 teaspoon ground ginger
- 1/4 teaspoon crushed red pepper flakes (optional)
- Salt and pepper to taste

PreparationTime: 20 minutes
Cook Time: 0 minutes
Total Time: 20 minutes
Serves: 4

Instructions:

1. In a large bowl, combine the shredded chicken, cabbage, carrots, bell pepper, and green onions.

2. In a small bowl, whisk together the rice vinegar, sesame oil, soy sauce, honey, ginger, and red pepper flakes (if using). Season with salt and pepper to taste.

3. Pour the sesame dressing over the salad and toss gently to coat.

4. Sprinkle the toasted sesame seeds over the top.

5. Serve the Asian chicken salad immediately.

This Asian-inspired salad is a great option for a menopause-friendly diet. The shredded chicken provides lean protein, while the vegetables offer fiber, vitamins, and minerals. The sesame dressing adds healthy fats and a delicious flavor. This salad is refreshing, satisfying, and packed with nutrients to support overall health during menopause.

33. Caprese Salad with Fresh Basil

Ingredients:

- 8 oz fresh mozzarella cheese, sliced
- 2 medium tomatoes, sliced
- 1/4 cup fresh basil leaves, torn or chopped
- 2 tablespoons balsamic glaze
- 1 tablespoon extra-virgin olive oil
- 1/4 teaspoon salt
- 1/8 teaspoon ground black pepper

PreparationTime: 10 minutes
Cook Time: 0 minutes
Total Time: 10 minutes
Serves: 4

Instructions:

1. Arrange the sliced mozzarella and tomatoes on a serving platter or individual plates.

2. Sprinkle the torn or chopped basil leaves over the top.

3. Drizzle the balsamic glaze and olive oil over the salad.

4. Season with salt and ground black pepper.

5. Serve immediately.

This classic Caprese salad is a great option for a menopause-friendly diet. The fresh mozzarella provides calcium, while the tomatoes are rich in lycopene, an antioxidant that may help reduce the risk of certain cancers. The basil adds flavor and anti-inflammatory properties. The balsamic glaze and olive oil provide healthy fats to help absorb the fat-soluble vitamins in the salad.

This simple yet flavorful salad is a refreshing and nutritious choice that can be enjoyed as a light main dish or a side salad. It's a great way to incorporate more plant-based foods into your diet during menopause.

34. Zucchini Noodles with Pesto and Cherry Tomatoes

Ingredients:

- 3 medium zucchini, spiralized or
  julienned into noodles
- 1/2 cup basil pesto (store-bought
  or homemade)
- 1 cup cherry tomatoes, halved
- 2 tablespoons toasted pine nuts
- 2 tablespoons grated Parmesan cheese (optional)
- Salt and pepper to taste

PreparationTime: 15 minutes
Cook Time: 5 minutes
Total Time: 20 minutes
Serves: 4

Instructions:

1. In a large skillet or wok, bring a small amount of water to a simmer over medium heat. Add the zucchini noodles and cook for 2-3 minutes, just until tender but still crisp. Drain and transfer to a large bowl.

2. Add the basil pesto to the zucchini noodles and toss gently to coat.

3. Stir in the halved cherry tomatoes, toasted pine nuts, and Parmesan cheese (if using). Season with salt and pepper to taste.

4. Serve the zucchini noodles with pesto and tomatoes immediately, while still warm.

This zucchini noodle dish is a great option for a menopause-friendly diet. Zucchini is low in calories and high in fiber, vitamins, and minerals. The basil pesto provides healthy fats from the olive oil and pine nuts, as well as antioxidants from the basil. The cherry tomatoes add a burst of vitamin C and lycopene. This colorful and flavorful meal is both nutritious and satisfying.

35. Beet and Goat Cheese Salad

Ingredients:

- 3 medium beets, peeled and cut into 1-inch cubes
- 1 tablespoon olive oil
- Salt and pepper to taste
- 4 cups mixed greens
 (such as spinach, arugula, kale)
- 1/2 cup crumbled goat cheese
- 2 tablespoons toasted walnuts
- 2 tablespoons balsamic vinegar
- 1 tablespoon honey

PreparationTime: 15 minutes
Cook Time: 30 minutes
Total Time: 45 minutes
Serves: 4

Instructions:

1. Preheat oven to 400°F. Toss the cubed beets with the olive oil and season with salt and pepper.

2. Spread the beets in a single layer on a baking sheet. Roast for 25-30 minutes, stirring halfway, until the beets are tender and lightly caramelized.

3. Allow the roasted beets to cool slightly.

4. In a large salad bowl, combine the mixed greens, roasted beets, crumbled goat cheese, and toasted walnuts.

5. In a small bowl, whisk together the balsamic vinegar and honey. Season with salt and pepper.

6. Drizzle the balsamic dressing over the salad and toss gently to coat.

7. Serve the beet and goat cheese salad immediately.

This beet and goat cheese salad is a great option for a menopause-friendly diet. Beets are rich in folate, manganese, and antioxidants, which can help support overall health during menopause. The goat cheese provides calcium and protein, while the walnuts add healthy fats and fiber. The balsamic vinegar and honey dressing adds flavor without too much added sugar. This colorful and nutrient-dense salad is both delicious and nourishing.

36. Tabbouleh with Fresh Parsley and Mint

Ingredients:

- 1 cup uncooked bulgur wheat
- 1 1/2 cups boiling water
- 1 cup chopped fresh parsley
- 1/2 cup chopped fresh mint
- 1 cup diced cucumber
- 1 cup diced tomatoes
- 1/2 cup diced red onion
- 2 tablespoons lemon juice
- 2 tablespoons extra-virgin olive oil
- 1/2 teaspoon ground cumin
- 1/4 teaspoon salt
- 1/4 teaspoon black pepper

PreparationTime: 20 minutes
Cook Time: 15 minutes
Total Time: 35 minutes
Serves: 4

Instructions:

1. In a medium bowl, combine the bulgur wheat and boiling water. Cover and let stand for 15 minutes, until the bulgur is tender and the water is absorbed.

2. Fluff the bulgur with a fork and transfer to a large serving bowl.

3. Add the chopped parsley, mint, cucumber, tomatoes, and red onion to the bowl with the bulgur.

4. In a small bowl, whisk together the lemon juice, olive oil, cumin, salt, and black pepper.

5. Pour the dressing over the tabbouleh salad and toss gently to combine.

6. Serve the tabbouleh salad chilled or at room temperature.

This tabbouleh salad is a great option for a menopause-friendly diet. The bulgur wheat provides complex carbohydrates and fiber, while the fresh herbs, vegetables, and lemon juice add vitamins, minerals, and antioxidants. The olive oil provides healthy fats to help absorb the fat-soluble nutrients. This refreshing and flavorful salad is a nutritious and satisfying choice during menopause.

37. Spicy Lentil Salad with Carrots and Cilantro

Ingredients:

- 1 cup dry brown or green lentils, rinsed
- 3 cups low-sodium vegetable broth
- 1 teaspoon ground cumin
- 1/2 teaspoon ground coriander
- 1/4 teaspoon cayenne pepper (or to taste)
- 1/4 teaspoon salt
- 2 carrots, peeled and grated
- 1/2 cup chopped fresh cilantro
- 2 tablespoons fresh lemon juice
- 1 tablespoon extra-virgin olive oil
- 1/4 teaspoon black pepper

PreparationTime: 15 minutes
Cook Time: 20 minutes
Total Time: 35 minutes
Serves: 4

Instructions:

1. In a medium saucepan, combine the lentils and vegetable broth. Bring to a boil over high heat.

2. Reduce heat to low, cover, and simmer for 15-20 minutes, until the lentils are tender. Drain any excess liquid.

3. Transfer the cooked lentils to a large bowl. Stir in the cumin, coriander, cayenne, and salt. Allow to cool slightly.

4. Add the grated carrots, chopped cilantro, lemon juice, olive oil, and black pepper. Toss to combine.

5. Serve the spicy lentil salad chilled or at room temperature.

This spicy lentil salad is a great option for a menopause-friendly diet. Lentils are an excellent source of plant-based protein, fiber, and complex carbohydrates. The carrots provide beta-carotene and other antioxidants, while the cilantro offers anti-inflammatory benefits. The lemon juice and olive oil add healthy fats to help absorb the fat-soluble nutrients. This flavorful and nutrient-dense salad is a satisfying and nourishing choice.

38. Turkey and Spinach Stuffed Peppers

Ingredients:

- 4 medium bell peppers,
halved lengthwise and seeded
- 1 lb ground turkey
- 1 cup cooked brown rice
- 2 cups fresh spinach, chopped
- 1/2 cup diced onion
- 2 cloves garlic, minced
- 1 teaspoon dried oregano
- 1/2 teaspoon ground cumin
- 1/4 teaspoon red pepper flakes (optional)
- 1/2 cup shredded mozzarella cheese
- Salt and pepper to taste

PreparationTime: 20 minutes
Cook Time: 30 minutes
Total Time: 50 minutes
Serves: 4

Instructions:

1. Preheat oven to 375°F. Place the bell pepper halves in a baking dish and set aside.

2. In a large skillet over medium heat, cook the ground turkey, breaking it up as it cooks, until no longer pink, about 5-7 minutes.

3. Add the onion and garlic to the skillet and cook for 2-3 minutes until fragrant.

4. Stir in the cooked brown rice, chopped spinach, oregano, cumin, and red pepper flakes (if using). Season with salt and pepper to taste.

5. Spoon the turkey and spinach mixture evenly into the bell pepper halves.

6. Top each stuffed pepper with a sprinkle of shredded mozzarella cheese.

7. Bake for 25-30 minutes, until the peppers are tender and the cheese is melted.

8. Serve the turkey and spinach stuffed peppers warm.

This recipe is a great option for a menopause-friendly diet. The bell peppers provide fiber, vitamins, and antioxidants, while the ground turkey offers lean protein. The spinach and brown rice add additional nutrients and complex carbohydrates. This dish is a balanced and satisfying meal that can help support overall health during menopause.

39. Mediterranean Farro Salad

Ingredients:

- 1 cup uncooked farro
- 2 cups low-sodium vegetable or chicken broth
- 1 cup cherry tomatoes, halved
- 1 cucumber, diced
- 1/2 cup crumbled feta cheese
- 1/4 cup kalamata olives, sliced
- 1/4 cup chopped fresh parsley
- 2 tablespoons chopped fresh basil
- 2 tablespoons lemon juice
- 1 tablespoon extra-virgin olive oil
- 1 teaspoon dried oregano
- 1/4 teaspoon salt
- 1/4 teaspoon black pepper

PreparationTime: 15 minutes
Cook Time: 20 minutes
Total Time: 35 minutes
Serves: 4

Instructions:

1. In a medium saucepan, combine the farro and broth. Bring to a boil over high heat, then reduce heat to low, cover, and simmer for 18-20 minutes, until the farro is tender. Drain any excess liquid and let cool slightly.

2. In a large bowl, combine the cooked farro, cherry tomatoes, cucumber, feta cheese, olives, parsley, and basil.

3. In a small bowl, whisk together the lemon juice, olive oil, oregano, salt, and black pepper.

4. Pour the dressing over the farro salad and toss gently to coat.

5. Serve the Mediterranean farro salad chilled or at room temperature.

This farro salad is a great option for a menopause-friendly diet. Farro is an ancient whole grain that provides fiber, protein, and complex carbohydrates. The vegetables, herbs, and olive oil provide antioxidants, vitamins, and healthy fats to support overall health during menopause. The feta cheese adds calcium, while the olives offer anti-inflammatory benefits. This refreshing and flavorful salad is a nutritious and satisfying choice.

40. Mixed Green Salad with Salmon and Lemon Dressing

Ingredients:

PreparationTime: 15 minutes
Cook Time: 10 minutes
Total Time: 25 minutes
Serves: 4

- 8 oz salmon fillet
- 1 tablespoon olive oil
- Salt and pepper to taste
- 6 cups mixed greens
 (such as spinach, arugula, kale)
- 1 cup cherry tomatoes, halved
- 1/2 cup sliced cucumber
- 2 tablespoons chopped fresh dill
- 2 tablespoons lemon juice
- 1 tablespoon Dijon mustard
- 1 tablespoon honey
- 1 tablespoon extra-virgin olive oil
- 1/4 teaspoon salt
- 1/8 teaspoon black pepper

Instructions:

1. Preheat oven to 400°F. Place the salmon fillet on a baking sheet, drizzle with 1 tablespoon olive oil, and season with salt and pepper.

2. Roast the salmon for 8-10 minutes, until cooked through and flaky. Allow to cool slightly, then flake the salmon into large chunks.

3. In a large salad bowl, combine the mixed greens, cherry tomatoes, cucumber, and chopped dill.

4. In a small bowl, whisk together the lemon juice, Dijon mustard, honey, 1 tablespoon olive oil, 1/4 teaspoon salt, and 1/8 teaspoon black pepper.

5. Add the flaked salmon to the salad and drizzle the lemon dressing over the top. Toss gently to coat. Serve the mixed green salad with salmon immediately.

This salmon salad is a great option for a menopause-friendly diet. Salmon is an excellent source of omega-3 fatty acids, which can help reduce inflammation. The mixed greens, tomatoes, and cucumber provide fiber, vitamins, and antioxidants. The lemon dressing adds a refreshing flavor and healthy fats to help absorb the fat-soluble nutrients. This nutrient-dense salad is a satisfying and nourishing meal.

41. Baked Salmon with Steamed Broccoli and Sweet Potatoes

Ingredients:

- 4 (6 oz) salmon fillets
- 1 tablespoon olive oil
- 1 teaspoon lemon pepper seasoning
- 1 lb broccoli florets
- 2 medium sweet potatoes, peeled and cubed
- 1 tablespoon unsalted butter
- Salt and pepper to taste

PreparationTime: 15 minutes
Cook Time: 30 minutes
Total Time: 45 minutes
Serves: 4

Instructions:

1. Preheat oven to 400°F. Line a baking sheet with parchment paper.

2. Place the salmon fillets on the prepared baking sheet. Drizzle with olive oil and sprinkle with lemon pepper seasoning.

3. Bake the salmon for 12-15 minutes, until it flakes easily with a fork.

4. While the salmon is baking, place the broccoli florets in a steamer basket over a pot of simmering water. Steam for 5-7 minutes, until tender-crisp.

5. In a separate pot, cover the cubed sweet potatoes with water. Bring to a boil, then reduce heat and simmer for 12-15 minutes, until the sweet potatoes are fork-tender.

6. Drain the sweet potatoes and toss with the butter. Season with salt and pepper to taste.

7. Serve the baked salmon fillets with the steamed broccoli and buttered sweet potatoes.

This balanced meal is an excellent choice for a menopause-friendly diet. Salmon is rich in omega-3 fatty acids, which can help reduce inflammation. Broccoli is a cruciferous vegetable that provides fiber, vitamins, and antioxidants. Sweet potatoes are a great source of complex carbohydrates, fiber, and beta-carotene. This nutrient-dense dinner is both satisfying and supportive of overall health during menopause.

42. Grilled Chicken with Quinoa and Roasted Vegetables

Ingredients:

- 4 (6 oz) boneless, skinless chicken breasts
- 1 tablespoon olive oil
- 1 teaspoon dried oregano
- 1/2 teaspoon garlic powder
- Salt and pepper to taste
- 1 cup uncooked quinoa, rinsed
- 2 cups low-sodium chicken or vegetable broth
- 1 medium zucchini, diced
- 1 medium yellow squash, diced
- 1 red bell pepper, diced
- 1 red onion, diced
- 2 tablespoons olive oil
- 1 teaspoon dried thyme
- 1/4 teaspoon cayenne pepper (optional)

PreparationTime: 20 minutes
Cook Time: 40 minutes
Total Time: 1 hour
Serves: 4

Instructions:

1. Preheat grill or grill pan to medium-high heat.

2. In a small bowl, combine the olive oil, oregano, garlic powder, salt, and pepper. Rub the mixture over the chicken breasts.

3. Grill the chicken for 5-7 minutes per side, until cooked through. Set aside and keep warm.

4. In a medium saucepan, combine the quinoa and broth. Bring to a boil, then reduce heat to low, cover, and simmer for 15-20 minutes, until quinoa is cooked.

5. Preheat oven to 400°F. Line a baking sheet with parchment paper.. In a large bowl, toss the diced zucchini, yellow squash, bell pepper, and onion with 2 tablespoons olive oil, thyme, and cayenne (if using). Season with salt and pepper.

7. Spread the vegetables in a single layer on the prepared baking sheet. Roast for 20-25 minutes, stirring halfway, until vegetables are tender and lightly browned. Serve the grilled chicken over the cooked quinoa, topped with the roasted vegetables.

This balanced meal is an excellent choice for a menopause-friendly diet. The grilled chicken provides lean protein, while the quinoa and roasted vegetables offer complex carbohydrates, fiber, and a variety of vitamins and minerals. This dish is both nutritious and satisfying.

43. Stir-Fried Tofu with Vegetables and Brown Rice

Ingredients:

Balanced Dinners

- 1 cup uncooked brown rice
- 2 cups low-sodium vegetable broth
- 1 block (14 oz) extra-firm tofu, drained and cubed
- 2 tablespoons low-sodium soy sauce
- 1 tablespoon sesame oil
- 1 tablespoon rice vinegar
- 1 teaspoon honey
- 1 tablespoon olive oil
- 2 cloves garlic, minced
- 1 inch piece fresh ginger, peeled and grated
- 1 red bell pepper, sliced
- 1 cup broccoli florets
- 1 cup sliced mushrooms
- 2 cups baby spinach
- 2 tablespoons toasted sesame seeds (optional)

PreparationTime: 20 minutes
Cook Time: 20 minutes
Total Time: 40 minutes
Serves: 4

Instructions:

1. In a medium saucepan, combine the brown rice and vegetable broth. Bring to a boil, then reduce heat to low, cover, and simmer for 18-20 minutes, until rice is tender. Fluff with a fork.

2. In a small bowl, whisk together the soy sauce, sesame oil, rice vinegar, and honey. Set aside.

3. Heat the olive oil in a large skillet or wok over medium-high heat. Add the garlic and ginger and cook for 1 minute, until fragrant.

4. Add the cubed tofu and cook for 2-3 minutes, until lightly browned on all sides.

5. Add the sliced bell pepper, broccoli, and mushrooms. Stir-fry for 5-7 minutes, until vegetables are tender-crisp.

6. Pour the soy sauce mixture over the tofu and vegetables and toss to coat.

7. Add the baby spinach and cook for 1-2 minutes, until wilted.

8. Serve the stir-fried tofu and vegetables over the cooked brown rice. Sprinkle with toasted sesame seeds, if desired.

This stir-fry dish is a great option for a menopause-friendly diet. Tofu provides plant-based protein, while the vegetables offer fiber, vitamins, and antioxidants. The brown rice is a complex carbohydrate that provides sustained energy. This flavorful and nutrient-dense meal is both satisfying and supportive of overall health during menopause.

44. Spaghetti Squash with Marinara Sauce and Ground Turkey

Ingredients:

- 1 medium spaghetti squash, halved lengthwise and seeded
- 1 lb ground turkey
- 1 tablespoon olive oil
- 1 onion, diced
- 3 cloves garlic, minced
- 1 (28 oz) can crushed tomatoes
- 2 tablespoons tomato paste
- 1 teaspoon dried oregano
- 1/2 teaspoon dried basil
- 1/4 teaspoon red pepper flakes (optional)
- Salt and pepper to taste
- 2 tablespoons grated Parmesan cheese (optional)
- 2 tablespoons chopped fresh parsley (optional)

PreparationTime: 15 minutes
Cook Time: 45 minutes
Total Time: 1 hour
Serves: 4

Instructions:

1. Preheat oven to 400°F. Place the spaghetti squash halves cut-side down on a baking sheet. Roast for 35-45 minutes, until tender when pierced with a fork.

2. In a large skillet, cook the ground turkey over medium-high heat, breaking it up as it cooks, until no longer pink, about 5-7 minutes. Transfer the cooked turkey to a plate and set aside.

3. In the same skillet, heat the olive oil over medium heat. Add the diced onion and sauté for 3-4 minutes until translucent.

4. Add the minced garlic and cook for 1 minute, until fragrant.

5. Stir in the crushed tomatoes, tomato paste, oregano, basil, and red pepper flakes (if using). Season with salt and pepper to taste.

6. Reduce heat to low and let the marinara sauce simmer for 10-15 minutes, stirring occasionally.

7. Add the cooked ground turkey back to the sauce and stir to combine.

8. Use a fork to shred the roasted spaghetti squash into strands. Divide the squash between 4 plates or bowls.

9. Top the spaghetti squash with the turkey marinara sauce. Sprinkle with Parmesan cheese and chopped parsley, if desired.

This spaghetti squash dish is a great option for a menopause-friendly diet. Spaghetti squash is low in calories and high in fiber, while the ground turkey provides lean protein. The marinara sauce adds antioxidants from the tomatoes. This meal is both nutritious and satisfying.

45. Baked Cod with Roasted Brussels Sprouts and Brown Rice

Ingredients:

- 4 (6 oz) cod fillets
- 1 tablespoon olive oil
- 1 teaspoon paprika
- 1/2 teaspoon garlic powder
- Salt and pepper to taste
- 1 lb Brussels sprouts, trimmed and halved
- 2 tablespoons olive oil
- 1 cup uncooked brown rice
- 2 cups low-sodium vegetable or chicken broth
- 2 tablespoons chopped fresh parsley (optional)

PreparationTime: 15 minutes
Cook Time: 35 minutes
Total Time: 50 minutes
Serves: 4

Instructions:

1. Preheat oven to 400°F. Line a baking sheet with parchment paper.

2. Place the cod fillets on the prepared baking sheet. Drizzle with 1 tablespoon olive oil and sprinkle with paprika, garlic powder, salt, and pepper.

3. In a large bowl, toss the Brussels sprouts with 2 tablespoons olive oil and season with salt and pepper.

4. Spread the Brussels sprouts in a single layer on a separate baking sheet.

5. Bake the cod and Brussels sprouts for 18-22 minutes, until the fish is opaque and flakes easily with a fork, and the Brussels sprouts are tender and lightly browned.

6. Meanwhile, in a medium saucepan, combine the brown rice and broth. Bring to a boil, then reduce heat to low, cover, and simmer for 18-20 minutes, until the rice is tender.

7. Fluff the cooked brown rice with a fork. Serve the baked cod over the brown rice, topped with the roasted Brussels sprouts. Garnish with chopped fresh parsley, if desired.

This balanced meal is an excellent choice for a menopause-friendly diet. The baked cod provides lean protein and omega-3 fatty acids, while the Brussels sprouts offer fiber, vitamins, and antioxidants. The brown rice is a complex carbohydrate that provides sustained energy. This nutritious and satisfying dish supports overall health during menopause.

46. Vegetable and Tofu Kebabs with Couscous

Ingredients:

- 1 block (14 oz) extra-firm tofu, cut into 1-inch cubes
- 1 red bell pepper, cut into 1-inch pieces
- 1 zucchini, cut into 1-inch slices
- 1 red onion, cut into 1-inch pieces
- 8 oz mushrooms, halved
- 2 tablespoons olive oil
- 1 teaspoon dried oregano
- 1/2 teaspoon garlic powder
- Salt and pepper to taste
- 1 cup uncooked whole wheat couscous
- 1 1/4 cups low-sodium vegetable broth
- 2 tablespoons chopped fresh parsley

PreparationTime: 20 minutes
Cook Time: 20 minutes
Total Time: 40 minutes
Serves: 4

Instructions:

1. Preheat grill or grill pan to medium-high heat.

2. In a large bowl, gently toss the tofu cubes, bell pepper, zucchini, onion, and mushrooms with the olive oil, oregano, garlic powder, salt, and pepper.

3. Thread the marinated vegetables and tofu onto skewers.

4. Grill the kebabs for 15-20 minutes, turning occasionally, until the vegetables are tender and the tofu is lightly charred.

5. Meanwhile, in a medium saucepan, bring the vegetable broth to a boil. Stir in the couscous, cover, and remove from heat. Let stand for 5-7 minutes, until the couscous is tender.

6. Fluff the cooked couscous with a fork and stir in the chopped parsley.

7. Serve the grilled vegetable and tofu kebabs over the parsley couscous.

This vegetarian kebab dish is a great option for a menopause-friendly diet. The tofu provides plant-based protein, while the vegetables offer fiber, vitamins, and antioxidants. The whole wheat couscous is a complex carbohydrate that provides sustained energy. This colorful and flavorful meal is both nutritious and satisfying.

47. Lemon Herb Chicken with Quinoa Salad

Ingredients:

Lemon Herb Chicken:
- 4 (6 oz) boneless, skinless chicken breasts
- 2 tablespoons olive oil
- 2 tablespoons lemon juice
- 1 tablespoon chopped fresh parsley
- 1 tablespoon chopped fresh thyme
- 1 teaspoon garlic powder
- Salt and pepper to taste

PreparationTime: 20 minutes
Cook Time: 30 minutes
Total Time: 50 minutes
Serves: 4

Quinoa Salad:
- 1 cup uncooked quinoa, rinsed
- 2 cups low-sodium chicken or vegetable broth
- 1 cup diced cucumber
- 1 cup cherry tomatoes, halved
- 1/2 cup crumbled feta cheese
- 2 tablespoons chopped fresh basil
- 2 tablespoons lemon juice
- 1 tablespoon olive oil
- 1/4 teaspoon salt
- 1/8 teaspoon black pepper

Instructions:

Lemon Herb Chicken:
1. Preheat oven to 400°F. Line a baking sheet with parchment paper.
2. In a shallow dish, combine the olive oil, lemon juice, parsley, thyme, garlic powder, salt, and pepper. Add the chicken breasts and turn to coat evenly.
3. Place the chicken on the prepared baking sheet and bake for 25-30 minutes, until the chicken is cooked through and reaches an internal temperature of 165°F.

Quinoa Salad:
1. In a medium saucepan, combine the quinoa and broth. Bring to a boil, then reduce heat to low, cover, and simmer for 15-20 minutes, until quinoa is cooked.
2. Fluff the quinoa with a fork and transfer to a large bowl. Allow to cool slightly.
3. Add the diced cucumber, cherry tomatoes, feta cheese, and chopped basil to the quinoa.
4. In a small bowl, whisk together the lemon juice, olive oil, salt, and pepper.
5. Pour the dressing over the quinoa salad and toss gently to combine.

Serve the lemon herb chicken alongside the quinoa salad.

This balanced meal is an excellent choice for a menopause-friendly diet. The lemon herb chicken provides lean protein, while the quinoa salad offers complex carbohydrates, fiber, and a variety of vitamins and minerals. The combination of flavors and nutrients makes this a satisfying and nourishing option.

48. Shrimp and Vegetable Stir-Fry

Ingredients:

- 1 lb raw shrimp, peeled and deveined
- 2 tablespoons low-sodium soy sauce
- 1 tablespoon rice vinegar
- 1 teaspoon sesame oil
- 1 tablespoon olive oil
- 3 cloves garlic, minced
- 1 inch piece fresh ginger, peeled and grated
- 1 red bell pepper, sliced
- 1 cup broccoli florets
- 1 cup snow peas
- 1 cup sliced mushrooms
- 2 cups cooked brown rice

PreparationTime: 15 minutes
Cook Time: 15 minutes
Total Time: 30 minutes
Serves: 4

Instructions:

1. In a small bowl, combine the soy sauce, rice vinegar, and sesame oil. Set aside.

2. Heat the olive oil in a large skillet or wok over medium-high heat.

3. Add the minced garlic and grated ginger and cook for 1 minute, until fragrant.

4. Add the shrimp and stir-fry for 2-3 minutes, until the shrimp start to turn pink.

5. Add the sliced bell pepper, broccoli florets, snow peas, and mushrooms. Stir-fry for 5-7 minutes, until the vegetables are tender-crisp.

6. Pour the soy sauce mixture over the shrimp and vegetables and toss to coat.

7. Serve the shrimp and vegetable stir-fry over the cooked brown rice.

This shrimp and vegetable stir-fry is a great option for a menopause-friendly diet. Shrimp provides lean protein and omega-3 fatty acids, while the vegetables offer fiber, vitamins, and antioxidants. The brown rice is a complex carbohydrate that provides sustained energy. This flavorful and nutrient-dense dish is both satisfying and supportive of overall health during menopause.

49. Black Bean and Sweet Potato Tacos

Ingredients:

- 2 medium sweet potatoes, peeled and diced
- 1 tablespoon olive oil
- 1 teaspoon chili powder
- 1/2 teaspoon ground cumin
- Salt and pepper to taste
- 1 (15 oz) can black beans, rinsed and drained
- 1/4 cup water
- 8 small whole wheat tortillas or taco shells
- 1 cup shredded red cabbage
- 1/2 cup diced avocado
- 2 tablespoons crumbled feta cheese
- 2 tablespoons chopped fresh cilantro

PreparationTime: 20 minutes
Cook Time: 25 minutes
Total Time: 45 minutes
Serves: 4 (2 tacos per serving)

Instructions:

1. Preheat oven to 400°F. Line a baking sheet with parchment paper.

2. In a large bowl, toss the diced sweet potatoes with the olive oil, chili powder, cumin, salt, and pepper. Spread the seasoned sweet potatoes in a single layer on the prepared baking sheet.

3. Roast the sweet potatoes for 20-25 minutes, stirring halfway, until tender and lightly browned.

4. In a medium saucepan, combine the black beans and water. Bring to a simmer over medium heat and cook for 5 minutes, until the beans are heated through.

5. Mash the black beans slightly with a fork or potato masher.

6. To assemble the tacos, spread a spoonful of the mashed black beans onto each tortilla or taco shell. Top with the roasted sweet potatoes, shredded cabbage, diced avocado, crumbled feta, and chopped cilantro.

7. Serve the black bean and sweet potato tacos immediately.

These vegetarian tacos are a great option for a menopause-friendly diet. The sweet potatoes provide complex carbohydrates, fiber, and beta-carotene, while the black beans offer plant-based protein and fiber. The avocado and feta add healthy fats and calcium. This colorful and flavorful meal is both nutritious and satisfying.

50. Baked Eggplant Parmesan

Ingredients:

- 1 large eggplant, sliced into 1/2-inch thick rounds
- 1 tablespoon olive oil
- 1 cup whole wheat breadcrumbs
- 1/2 cup grated Parmesan cheese
- 1 teaspoon dried oregano
- 1/2 teaspoon garlic powder
- 1/4 teaspoon salt
- 1/4 teaspoon black pepper
- 1 (24 oz) jar marinara sauce
- 1 cup shredded part-skim mozzarella cheese

PreparationTime: 30 minutes
Cook Time: 40 minutes
Total Time: 1 hour 10 minutes
Serves: 4

Instructions:

1. Preheat oven to 375°F. Lightly grease a 9x13 inch baking dish.

2. Brush both sides of the eggplant slices with the olive oil and place them in a single layer on a baking sheet.

3. In a shallow bowl, combine the breadcrumbs, Parmesan cheese, oregano, garlic powder, salt, and pepper.

4. Dip the eggplant slices into the breadcrumb mixture, pressing gently to help it adhere.

5. Arrange the breaded eggplant slices in a single layer in the prepared baking dish.

6. Spread the marinara sauce evenly over the eggplant slices.

7. Sprinkle the shredded mozzarella cheese over the top.

8. Bake for 35-40 minutes, until the eggplant is tender and the cheese is melted and bubbly.

9. Let the eggplant parmesan cool for 5 minutes before serving.

This baked eggplant parmesan is a delicious and healthier version of the classic dish. Eggplant is a great source of fiber, vitamins, and antioxidants. The whole wheat breadcrumbs and reduced-fat cheese keep this meal lighter and more menopause-friendly. Serve it with a fresh green salad for a complete and nourishing dinner.

51. Grilled Steak with Asparagus and Quinoa

Ingredients:

- 1 lb flank steak
- 2 tablespoons olive oil, divided
- 1 teaspoon garlic powder
- 1 teaspoon dried oregano
- Salt and pepper to taste
- 1 lb asparagus, trimmed
- 1 cup uncooked quinoa, rinsed
- 2 cups low-sodium chicken or vegetable broth
- 2 tablespoons chopped fresh parsley

PreparationTime: 20 minutes
Cook Time: 25 minutes
Total Time: 45 minutes
Serves: 4

Instructions:

1. Preheat grill or grill pan to medium-high heat.

2. In a shallow dish, combine 1 tablespoon of the olive oil, garlic powder, oregano, salt, and pepper. Add the flank steak and turn to coat both sides.

3. Grill the steak for 4-6 minutes per side, until it reaches your desired doneness. Transfer to a cutting board and let rest for 5 minutes before slicing against the grain.

4. In a large bowl, toss the asparagus with the remaining 1 tablespoon of olive oil and season with salt and pepper.

5. Grill the asparagus for 5-7 minutes, turning occasionally, until tender-crisp.

6. In a medium saucepan, combine the quinoa and broth. Bring to a boil, then reduce heat to low, cover, and simmer for 15-20 minutes, until the quinoa is cooked.

7. Fluff the quinoa with a fork and stir in the chopped parsley.

8. Serve the grilled steak slices alongside the grilled asparagus and quinoa.

This balanced meal is an excellent choice for a menopause-friendly diet. The grilled steak provides lean protein, while the asparagus offers fiber, vitamins, and antioxidants. The quinoa is a complete protein and a source of complex carbohydrates. This nutritious and satisfying dish supports overall health during menopause.

52. Moroccan Chickpea Stew

Ingredients:

- 2 tablespoons olive oil
- 1 onion, diced
- 3 cloves garlic, minced
- 1 tablespoon grated fresh ginger
- 1 teaspoon ground cumin
- 1 teaspoon ground coriander
- 1 teaspoon paprika
- 1/4 teaspoon cayenne pepper (optional)
- 1 (15 oz) can diced tomatoes
- 1 (15 oz) can chickpeas, rinsed and drained
- 1 cup low-sodium vegetable broth
- 1 cup chopped cauliflower florets
- 1 cup chopped sweet potato
- 1/4 cup chopped fresh cilantro
- Salt and pepper to taste
- Cooked quinoa or brown rice, for serving

PreparationTime: 20 minutes
Cook Time: 30 minutes
Total Time: 50 minutes
Serves: 4

Instructions:

1. In a large pot or Dutch oven, heat the olive oil over medium heat. Add the diced onion and sauté for 3-4 minutes until translucent.

2. Add the minced garlic and grated ginger. Cook for 1 minute, until fragrant.

3. Stir in the cumin, coriander, paprika, and cayenne (if using). Cook for 1 minute to toast the spices.

4. Pour in the diced tomatoes, chickpeas, and vegetable broth. Bring to a simmer.

5. Add the chopped cauliflower and sweet potato. Reduce heat to low, cover, and simmer for 20-25 minutes, until the vegetables are tender.

6. Remove from heat and stir in the chopped cilantro. Season with salt and pepper to taste. Serve the Moroccan chickpea stew over cooked quinoa or brown rice.

This flavorful Moroccan-inspired stew is a great option for a menopause-friendly diet. Chickpeas provide plant-based protein and fiber, while the vegetables offer a variety of vitamins, minerals, and antioxidants. The warm spices add depth of flavor without excessive sodium or sugar. This nourishing and satisfying dish is perfect for a comforting meal.

53. Roasted Chicken with Root Vegetables

Ingredients:

- 1 whole chicken (3-4 lbs),
cut into 8 pieces (breasts, thighs, legs, wings)
- 2 tablespoons olive oil
- 1 teaspoon dried thyme
- 1 teaspoon dried rosemary
- 1 teaspoon garlic powder
- Salt and pepper to taste
- 2 medium sweet potatoes, peeled and cubed
- 2 medium carrots, peeled and cut into 1-inch pieces
- 1 medium parsnip, peeled and cut into 1-inch pieces
- 1 medium red onion, cut into wedges
- 2 tablespoons chopped fresh parsley (optional)

PreparationTime: 20 minutes
Cook Time: 1 hour
Total Time: 1 hour 20 minutes
Serves: 4

Instructions:

1. Preheat oven to 400°F. Line a large baking sheet with parchment paper.

2. Pat the chicken pieces dry with paper towels and place them in a large bowl. Drizzle with the olive oil and sprinkle with the thyme, rosemary, garlic powder, salt, and pepper. Toss to coat the chicken evenly.

3. Arrange the chicken pieces skin-side up on the prepared baking sheet.

4. In a separate bowl, toss the cubed sweet potatoes, carrot pieces, parsnip pieces, and onion wedges with a drizzle of olive oil and a pinch of salt and pepper.

5. Spread the seasoned root vegetables around the chicken pieces on the baking sheet.

6. Roast for 55-60 minutes, until the chicken is cooked through (165°F internal temperature) and the vegetables are tender.

7. Transfer the chicken and roasted vegetables to a serving platter. Sprinkle with the chopped fresh parsley, if desired. Serve the roasted chicken and vegetables immediately.

This one-pan roasted chicken and vegetable dish is a great option for a menopause-friendly diet. The chicken provides lean protein, while the root vegetables offer complex carbohydrates, fiber, and a variety of vitamins and minerals. This satisfying and nutritious meal is easy to prepare and perfect for a comforting dinner.

54. Quinoa Stuffed Bell Peppers

Ingredients:

- 4 bell peppers (any color)
- 1 cup cooked quinoa
- 1 (15 oz) can black beans, drained and rinsed
- 1 cup diced tomatoes
- 1/2 cup diced onion
- 2 cloves garlic, minced
- 1 tsp cumin
- 1 tsp chili powder
- 1/4 tsp cayenne pepper (optional)
- Salt and pepper to taste
- 1 cup shredded cheese (cheddar, Monterey jack, etc.)

PreparationTime: 15 minutes
Cook Time: 30 minutes
Total Time: 45 minutes
Serves: 4

Instructions:

1. Preheat oven to 375°F. Cut the tops off the bell peppers and remove the seeds and membranes. Place the peppers in a baking dish.

2. In a bowl, mix together the cooked quinoa, black beans, diced tomatoes, onion, garlic, cumin, chili powder, cayenne (if using), salt and pepper.

3. Stuff the quinoa mixture into the hollowed out bell peppers, packing it in tightly.

4. Top each stuffed pepper with shredded cheese.

5. Bake for 25-30 minutes, until the peppers are tender and the cheese is melted and bubbly.

6. Serve hot. Enjoy!

 details!

55. Spinach and Feta Stuffed Chicken Breasts

Ingredients:

- 4 boneless, skinless chicken breasts
- 2 cups fresh spinach, chopped
- 1/2 cup crumbled feta cheese
- 2 cloves garlic, minced
- 1 tbsp olive oil
- 1 tsp dried oregano
- Salt and pepper to taste

PreparationTime: 20 minutes
Cook Time: 30 minutes
Total Time: 50 minutes
Serves: 4

Instructions:

1. Preheat oven to 375°F. Lightly grease a baking dish.

2. In a bowl, mix together the chopped spinach, feta cheese, garlic, oregano, salt and pepper.

3. Slice each chicken breast horizontally to create a pocket. Stuff each pocket with the spinach and feta mixture, dividing it evenly.

4. Place the stuffed chicken breasts in the prepared baking dish. Drizzle the tops with olive oil.

5. Bake for 25-30 minutes, until the chicken is cooked through and the internal temperature reaches 165°F.

6. Serve the spinach and feta stuffed chicken breasts warm. Enjoy!

This recipe is great for a menopause diet as it is:
- High in protein from the chicken
- Contains healthy fats from the olive oil and feta
- Provides fiber and nutrients from the spinach
- Avoids processed ingredients or added sugars

The spinach and feta filling also provides calcium, which is important for bone health during menopause. modifications!

56. Lentil and Vegetable Shepherd's Pie

Ingredients:

Balanced Dinners

Filling:
- 1 cup brown or green lentils, rinsed
- 3 cups vegetable broth
- 1 tbsp olive oil
- 1 onion, diced
- 3 carrots, peeled and diced
- 2 celery stalks, diced
- 3 cloves garlic, minced
- 1 tsp dried thyme
- 1 tsp dried rosemary
- Salt and pepper to taste

PreparationTime: 30 minutes
Cook Time: 45 minutes
Total Time: 1 hour 15 minutes
Serves: 6

Topping:
- 3 lbs russet or Yukon Gold potatoes, peeled and cut into 1-inch chunks
- 1/4 cup unsweetened almond milk
- 2 tbsp olive oil
- 1/2 tsp salt

Instructions:

1. Preheat oven to 375°F. Grease a 9x13 inch baking dish.

2. In a saucepan, combine the lentils and vegetable broth. Bring to a boil, then reduce heat and simmer for 20-25 minutes, until lentils are tender. Drain any excess liquid.

3. In a large skillet, heat the olive oil over medium heat. Add the onion, carrots, celery and garlic. Sauté for 5-7 minutes until vegetables are softened.

4. Stir the cooked lentils, thyme, rosemary, salt and pepper into the vegetable mixture. Spread evenly into the prepared baking dish.

5. In a large pot, cover the potato chunks with water. Bring to a boil and cook for 15-20 minutes until very tender. Drain and return to the pot.

6. Mash the potatoes with the almond milk, olive oil and salt until smooth and creamy.

7. Spread the mashed potatoes evenly over the lentil filling.

8. Bake for 30-35 minutes, until the potatoes are lightly browned on top.

9. Let stand for 5-10 minutes before serving.

Enjoy your hearty Lentil and Vegetable Shepherd's Pie!

57. Baked Halibut with Quinoa Pilaf

Ingredients:

Quinoa Pilaf:
- 1 cup uncooked quinoa, rinsed
- 2 cups low-sodium vegetable or chicken broth
- 1 tbsp olive oil
- 1 onion, diced
- 2 cloves garlic, minced
- 1 cup diced bell pepper
- 1 cup diced zucchini
- 2 tbsp chopped fresh parsley
- Salt and pepper to taste

Baked Halibut:
- 4 (6 oz) halibut fillets
- 2 tbsp olive oil
- 1 tsp lemon zest
- 2 tbsp lemon juice
- 2 tbsp chopped fresh dill
- Salt and pepper to taste

PreparationTime: 20 minutes
Cook Time: 30 minutes
Total Time: 50 minutes
Serves: 4

Instructions:

1. Preheat oven to 400°F. Grease a baking dish.

2. In a medium saucepan, combine the quinoa and broth. Bring to a boil, then reduce heat, cover and simmer for 15-20 minutes until quinoa is tender.

3. In a skillet, heat the olive oil over medium heat. Add the onion, garlic, bell pepper and zucchini. Sauté for 5-7 minutes until vegetables are softened.

4. Fluff the cooked quinoa with a fork and stir in the sautéed vegetables and parsley. Season with salt and pepper.

5. Place the halibut fillets in the prepared baking dish. Drizzle with olive oil and sprinkle with lemon zest, lemon juice, dill, salt and pepper.

6. Bake for 15-20 minutes, until the halibut is opaque and flakes easily with a fork. Serve the baked halibut over the quinoa pilaf. Enjoy!

This recipe is great for a menopause diet as it is:
- High in protein from the halibut
- Contains healthy fats from the olive oil and quinoa
- Provides fiber and nutrients from the vegetables
- Avoids processed ingredients or added sugars

58. Turkey Meatballs with Zucchini Noodles

Ingredients:

Balanced Dinners

Meatballs:
- 1 lb ground turkey
- 1/2 cup breadcrumbs
- 1 egg
- 2 cloves garlic, minced
- 1/4 cup grated Parmesan cheese
- 2 tbsp chopped fresh parsley
- 1 tsp dried oregano
- 1/2 tsp salt
- 1/4 tsp black pepper

PreparationTime: 25 minutes
Cook Time: 30 minutes
Total Time: 55 minutes
Serves: 4

Zucchini Noodles:
- 4 medium zucchinis, spiralized or julienned
- 2 tbsp olive oil
- 2 cloves garlic, minced
- 1 (24 oz) jar marinara sauce
- 1/4 cup shredded basil leaves

Instructions:

1. Preheat oven to 400°F. Line a baking sheet with parchment paper.

2. In a large bowl, combine all the meatball ingredients and mix well. Roll the mixture into 1-inch meatballs and place them on the prepared baking sheet.

3. Bake the meatballs for 20-25 minutes, until cooked through.

4. While the meatballs are baking, heat the olive oil in a large skillet over medium heat. Add the garlic and sauté for 1 minute until fragrant.

5. Add the spiralized or julienned zucchini noodles to the skillet. Sauté for 3-5 minutes, until the zucchini is tender but still has some bite.

6. Pour the marinara sauce over the zucchini noodles and stir to coat. Simmer for 2-3 minutes.

7. Serve the zucchini noodles topped with the baked turkey meatballs and garnished with fresh basil.

Enjoy your healthy and delicious Turkey Meatballs with Zucchini Noodles!

59. Chickpea and Spinach Curry

Ingredients:

- 1 tbsp olive oil
- 1 onion, diced
- 3 cloves garlic, minced
- 1 tbsp grated fresh ginger
- 1 tsp ground cumin
- 1 tsp ground coriander
- 1 tsp garam masala
- 1/2 tsp turmeric
- 1/4 tsp cayenne pepper (optional)
- 1 (15 oz) can chickpeas, drained and rinsed
- 1 (14 oz) can diced tomatoes
- 1 cup low-sodium vegetable broth
- 5 oz fresh spinach, chopped
- 1/4 cup full-fat coconut milk
- Salt and pepper to taste
- Chopped cilantro for garnish

PreparationTime: 15 minutes
Cook Time: 25 minutes
Total Time: 40 minutes
Serves: 4

Instructions:

1. In a large skillet, heat the olive oil over medium heat. Add the onion and sauté for 3-4 minutes until translucent.

2. Add the garlic, ginger, cumin, coriander, garam masala, turmeric and cayenne (if using). Cook for 1 minute, stirring constantly, until fragrant.

3. Stir in the chickpeas, diced tomatoes and vegetable broth. Bring to a simmer and cook for 10 minutes.

4. Add the chopped spinach and coconut milk. Simmer for 5 more minutes, until the spinach is wilted and the sauce has thickened slightly.

5. Season with salt and pepper to taste.

6. Serve the chickpea and spinach curry over basmati rice or with naan bread. Garnish with chopped cilantro.

This curry is an excellent choice for a menopause diet as it is:
- High in protein and fiber from the chickpeas
- Rich in iron, calcium and other nutrients from the spinach
- Contains healthy fats from the coconut milk
- Avoids processed ingredients or added sugars

The spices also provide anti-inflammatory benefits. Feel free to adjust the heat level to your preference. Enjoy!

60. Grilled Salmon with Mango Salsa and Brown Rice

Ingredients:

Mango Salsa:
- 1 ripe mango, diced
- 1/2 red onion, finely chopped
- 1 jalapeño, seeded and minced
- 1/4 cup chopped fresh cilantro
- 2 tbsp lime juice
- 1/4 tsp salt

the new menopause diet cookbook- 4 (6 oz) salmon fillets
- 2 tbsp olive oil
- 1 tsp chili powder
- 1 tsp ground cumin
- Salt and pepper to taste
- 2 cups cooked brown rice

Balanced Dinners

PreparationTime: 20 minutes
Cook Time: 30 minutes
Total Time: 50 minutes
Serves: 4

Instructions:
1. Preheat grill or grill pan to medium-high heat.

2. In a bowl, combine all the mango salsa ingredients and mix well. Set aside.

3. Pat the salmon fillets dry and brush with olive oil. Season with chili powder, cumin, salt and pepper.

4. Grill the salmon for 4-5 minutes per side, until cooked through and flakes easily with a fork. Serve the grilled salmon fillets over a bed of brown rice, topped with the fresh mango salsa.

This dish is an excellent choice for a menopause diet for a few reasons:

- Salmon is high in omega-3 fatty acids, which can help reduce inflammation.
- Mangoes are a good source of vitamins C and A, which are important for skin and immune health.
- Brown rice provides complex carbs, fiber, and B vitamins.
- The overall meal is balanced with lean protein, healthy fats, and nutrient-dense produce.

Feel free to adjust the spices or salsa ingredients to your taste. Enjoy your Grilled Salmon with Mango Salsa and Brown Rice!

61. Carrot Sticks with Hummus

Ingredients:

Hummus:
- 1 (15 oz) can chickpeas, drained and rinsed
- 2 tbsp tahini
- 2 tbsp fresh lemon juice
- 2 cloves garlic, minced
- 2 tbsp olive oil
- 1/4 tsp ground cumin
- 1/4 tsp paprika
- Salt and pepper to taste

PreparationTime: 10 minutes
Total Time: 10 minutes
Serves: 4

Carrot Sticks:
- 4-5 medium carrots, peeled and cut into sticks

Instructions:

1. In a food processor, combine all the hummus ingredients. Blend until smooth and creamy. Taste and adjust seasoning as needed.

2. Transfer the hummus to a serving bowl.

3. Wash and peel the carrots. Cut them into long, thin sticks.

4. Arrange the carrot sticks around the bowl of hummus.

5. Serve the carrot sticks with the homemade hummus for dipping.

This snack is an excellent choice for a menopause diet for a few reasons:

- Chickpeas in the hummus are high in protein, fiber, and complex carbs, which can help stabilize blood sugar levels.
- Carrots are rich in beta-carotene, an antioxidant that can help support skin and eye health.
- Tahini provides healthy fats and minerals like calcium, which is important for bone health during menopause.
- The overall dish is low in calories, sodium, and added sugars, making it a nutritious and satisfying snack.

Feel free to adjust the hummus recipe to your taste preferences. Enjoy your Carrot Sticks with Homemade Hummus!

62. Apple Slices with Almond Butter

Ingredients:

- 1 medium apple, cored and sliced
- 2 tbsp all-natural almond butter

Instructions:

1. Wash and slice the apple into thin wedges or slices.

2. Arrange the apple slices on a plate or small board.

3. Scoop the almond butter into a small bowl or ramekin.

4. Serve the apple slices alongside the almond butter for dipping.

This simple snack is an excellent choice for a menopause diet for a few reasons:

- Apples are a good source of fiber, which can help regulate digestion and blood sugar levels.
- Almond butter provides healthy fats, protein, and minerals like magnesium that are important during menopause.
- The combination of the crisp apple and creamy almond butter makes for a satisfying and nutritious snack.

Some additional tips:

- Choose a crisp, tart apple variety like Honeycrisp or Granny Smith.
- Look for an almond butter with no added sugars or oils.
- You can also sprinkle a pinch of cinnamon over the apple slices for extra flavor.

This snack is quick, easy, and portable, making it a great option for a healthy menopause-friendly treat. Enjoy!

Sides and Snacks

PreparationTime: 5 minutes
Total Time: 5 minutes
Serves: 1

63. Greek Yogurt with Honey and Walnuts

Ingredients:

- 1 cup plain Greek yogurt
- 1 tbsp raw honey
- 2 tbsp chopped walnuts

PreparationTime: 5 minutes
Total Time: 5 minutes
Serves: 1

Instructions:

1. Scoop the Greek yogurt into a serving bowl or container.

2. Drizzle the honey over the top of the yogurt.

3. Sprinkle the chopped walnuts over the honey.

4. Serve immediately.

This simple yogurt parfait is an excellent choice for a menopause diet for several reasons:

- Greek yogurt is high in protein, which can help maintain muscle mass and bone health.
- Honey provides natural sweetness and contains antioxidants that may help reduce inflammation.
- Walnuts are a great source of omega-3 fatty acids, which can help support brain and heart health.

Some additional tips:

- Choose a full-fat or 2% Greek yogurt for more creaminess and healthy fats.
- Look for raw, unprocessed honey for maximum nutritional benefits.
- You can also add a sprinkle of cinnamon or a handful of fresh berries for extra flavor and nutrients.

This yogurt parfait makes for a quick, satisfying, and nutrient-dense snack or light breakfast. The combination of protein, healthy fats, and natural sweetness makes it a great choice for managing menopause symptoms. Enjoy!

64. Handful of Walnuts

Ingredients:

- 1 oz (about 14 halves) raw, unsalted walnuts

Preparation

Instructions:
1. Measure out 1 oz (approximately a handful) of raw, unsalted walnuts.

2. Enjoy the walnuts as a healthy snack.

Nutritional Benefits:
- High in omega-3 fatty acids, which can help reduce inflammation and alleviate menopause symptoms

- Rich in antioxidants like ellagic acid and gamma-tocopherol, which may help reduce cancer risk

- Good source of magnesium, copper, and manganese - important minerals for bone health during menopause

- Promotes heart health with healthy fats, fiber, and plant sterols

- Contains melatonin to help regulate sleep cycles

Tips:
- Choose raw, unsalted walnuts for maximum nutritional benefits.

- Portion out 1 oz (about a handful) for a satisfying snack.

- You can also add walnuts to salads, yogurt, oatmeal, or baked goods.

Walnuts are an excellent, nutrient-dense snack choice for women going through menopause. Enjoy a handful daily as part of a healthy diet.

65. Sliced Bell Peppers with Guacamole

Ingredients:

Guacamole:
- 2 ripe avocados, pitted and diced
- 1/4 cup diced red onion
- 1 jalapeño, seeded and minced (optional)
- 2 tbsp chopped fresh cilantro
- 2 tbsp lime juice
- 1/2 tsp salt

Sliced Bell Peppers:
- 2 bell peppers (any color), sliced into strips

PreparationTime: 15 minutes
Total Time: 15 minutes
Serves: 4

Instructions:

1. In a medium bowl, gently mix together all the guacamole ingredients until well combined. Taste and adjust seasoning as needed.

2. Arrange the sliced bell pepper strips on a serving platter or plate.

3. Scoop the guacamole into a small bowl and place it in the center of the plate with the bell pepper slices around it.

4. Serve the sliced bell peppers with the homemade guacamole for dipping.

This healthy snack is a great option for a menopause diet for a few reasons:

- Bell peppers are an excellent source of vitamin C, which can help support the immune system during menopause.
- Avocados in the guacamole provide healthy monounsaturated fats that can help reduce inflammation.
- The combination of the crunchy peppers and creamy guacamole makes for a satisfying and nutrient-dense snack.

You can adjust the spice level of the guacamole by including or omitting the jalapeño. Feel free to experiment with different colored bell peppers as well.

Enjoy your Sliced Bell Peppers with Homemade Guacamole!

66. Fresh Fruit Salad

Ingredients:

- 2 cups diced fresh pineapple
- 2 cups diced fresh mango
- 2 cups diced fresh strawberries
- 1 cup diced fresh kiwi
- 1 cup diced fresh grapes
- 2 tablespoons fresh lime juice
- 1 tablespoon honey (optional)
- Mint leaves for garnish (optional)

PreparationTime: 15 minutes
Cook Time: 0 minutes
Total Time: 45 minutes (including chilling time)
Serves: 6-8 servings

Instructions:

1. In a large bowl, combine the diced pineapple, mango, strawberries, kiwi, and grapes.

2. Drizzle the lime juice over the fruit and gently toss to coat.

3. If desired, drizzle the honey over the fruit and toss again to combine.

4. Cover and refrigerate for at least 30 minutes to allow the flavors to meld.

5. Just before serving, give the salad another gentle toss.

6. Garnish with fresh mint leaves, if desired.

Serve chilled. This fresh fruit salad is a delicious and healthy dessert or side dish. The combination of tropical and seasonal fruits creates a vibrant and refreshing salad.

67. Edamame with Sea Salt

Ingredients:

- 1 lb fresh edamame in the pod
- 1 tablespoon coarse sea salt

Instructions:

PreparationTime: 5 minutes
Cook Time: 5 minutes
Total Time: 10 minutes
Serves: 4 servings

1. Bring a large pot of salted water to a boil.

2. Add the edamame pods and cook for 5 minutes, or until the beans are tender.

3. Drain the edamame and transfer to a serving bowl.

4. Sprinkle the coarse sea salt over the hot edamame and toss to coat evenly.

5. Serve the edamame warm, with the pods intact. Provide small dishes for discarding the empty pods.

Tips:
- You can adjust the amount of salt to taste.
- Edamame can also be served chilled or at room temperature.
- For a flavor twist, try adding a squeeze of lemon or lime juice.

Edamame is a healthy and delicious snack or appetizer. The combination of the tender, slightly sweet beans and the crunchy sea salt makes for a tasty and satisfying treat.

68. Cottage Cheese with Sliced Peaches

Ingredients:

- 1/2 cup low-fat or non-fat cottage cheese
- 1 medium fresh peach, sliced
- 1 teaspoon honey (optional)

Instructions:

1. Place the cottage cheese in a small bowl.

2. Arrange the sliced peaches on top of the cottage cheese.

3. If desired, drizzle the honey over the peaches and cottage cheese.

Nutritional Benefits for Menopause:
- Cottage cheese is a good source of protein, which can help maintain muscle mass during menopause.

- Peaches are rich in vitamins, minerals, and antioxidants, which can help support overall health during the menopausal transition.

- Honey can provide a natural sweetness without the added sugar, which is important for managing blood sugar levels.

This simple and refreshing dish is a great option for a healthy snack or light meal during menopause. The combination of the creamy cottage cheese and the sweet, juicy peaches provides a satisfying and nutritious treat.

PreparationTime: 5 minutes
Cook Time: 0 minutes
Total Time: 5 minutes
Serves: 1 serving

69. Celery Sticks with Peanut Butter

Ingredients:

- 2-3 celery stalks, cut into 4-inch sticks
- 2 tablespoons natural, unsweetened peanut butter

Nutritional Benefits for Menopause:

PreparationTime: 5 minutes
Cook Time: 0 minutes
Total Time: 5 minutes
Serves: 1 serving

- Celery is a low-calorie, high-fiber vegetable that can help with weight management during menopause.

- Peanut butter is a good source of protein, which can help maintain muscle mass and support overall health.

- The combination of the crunchy celery and the creamy peanut butter provides a satisfying and nutrient-dense snack.

Instructions:

1. Wash the celery stalks and cut them into 4-inch sticks.

2. Spread the peanut butter evenly onto the celery sticks.

Tips:
- Choose a natural, unsweetened peanut butter to avoid added sugars.

- You can also use other nut or seed butters, such as almond butter or sunflower seed butter, for variety.

- For extra flavor, you can sprinkle a pinch of cinnamon or a drizzle of honey on top of the peanut butter.

This simple and nutritious snack is a great option for a menopause-friendly diet. The combination of the fiber-rich celery and the protein-packed peanut butter can help keep you feeling full and satisfied between meals.

70. Roasted Chickpeas with Spices

Ingredients:

- 1 (15 oz) can chickpeas, drained and rinsed
- 1 tablespoon olive oil
- 1 teaspoon ground cumin
- 1 teaspoon paprika
- 1/2 teaspoon garlic powder
- 1/4 teaspoon cayenne pepper (optional)
- 1/4 teaspoon salt

Sides and Snacks

PreparationTime: 10 minutes
Cook Time: 25 minutes
Total Time: 35 minutes
Serves: 4 servings

Nutritional Benefits for Menopause:
- Chickpeas are a good source of plant-based protein, which can help maintain muscle mass during menopause.
- The spices used in this recipe, such as cumin and paprika, are rich in antioxidants that can help support overall health.
- The combination of protein, fiber, and healthy fats from the chickpeas and olive oil can help with weight management and blood sugar regulation during menopause.

Instructions:

1. Preheat your oven to 400°F (200°C).

2. Drain and rinse the chickpeas, then pat them dry with a paper towel or clean kitchen towel.

3. In a medium-sized bowl, toss the chickpeas with the olive oil, cumin, paprika, garlic powder, cayenne pepper (if using), and salt until they are evenly coated.

4. Spread the seasoned chickpeas in a single layer on a baking sheet lined with parchment paper.

5. Roast the chickpeas in the preheated oven for 20-25 minutes, stirring halfway, until they are crispy and golden brown.

6. Remove the roasted chickpeas from the oven and let them cool for a few minutes before serving.

Enjoy the roasted chickpeas as a healthy snack or add them to salads, soups, or other dishes. The spices can be adjusted to your taste preferences.

71. Cucumber Slices with Tzatziki

Ingredients:

Sides and Snacks

- 1 large cucumber, sliced into thin rounds
- 1 cup plain Greek yogurt
- 1 clove garlic, minced
- 1 tablespoon fresh lemon juice
- 1 tablespoon chopped fresh dill
(or 1 teaspoon dried dill)
- 1/4 teaspoon salt
- 1/4 teaspoon ground black pepper

PreparationTime: 10 minutes
Cook Time: 0 minutes
Total Time: 10 minutes
Serves: 4 servings

Nutritional Benefits for Menopause:
- Cucumbers are a low-calorie, high-fiber vegetable that can help with hydration and weight management during menopause.

- Greek yogurt is a good source of protein, which can help maintain muscle mass.

- The combination of the cooling cucumber and the creamy, tangy tzatziki dip provides a refreshing and satisfying snack.

- The fresh dill and lemon juice in the tzatziki are rich in antioxidants that can support overall health during the menopausal transition.

Instructions:

1. Slice the cucumber into thin rounds and set aside.

2. In a small bowl, mix together the Greek yogurt, minced garlic, lemon juice, chopped dill (or dried dill), salt, and black pepper until well combined.

3. Serve the cucumber slices with the tzatziki dip on the side. You can also top the cucumber slices with a small spoonful of the tzatziki.

Tips:
- For extra flavor, you can add a pinch of cumin or a drizzle of olive oil to the tzatziki.
- Adjust the amount of garlic, lemon, and dill to your personal taste preferences.
- This snack can also be served as a healthy appetizer or side dish.

Enjoy this refreshing and nutritious snack during your menopause journey!

72. Mixed Nuts and Seeds

Ingredients:

- 1/4 cup raw almonds
- 1/4 cup raw walnuts
- 1/4 cup raw pumpkin seeds (pepitas)
- 1/4 cup raw sunflower seeds
- 1 tablespoon chia seeds
- 1 tablespoon ground flaxseeds
- 1/4 teaspoon ground cinnamon (optional)
- 1/8 teaspoon sea salt (optional)

PreparationTime: 5 minutes
Cook Time: 0 minutes
Total Time: 5 minutes
Serves: 4 servings

Nutritional Benefits for Menopause:
- Nuts and seeds are rich in healthy fats, protein, fiber, and a variety of vitamins and minerals that can support overall health during menopause.
- Almonds and walnuts are good sources of magnesium, which can help with bone health and muscle function.
- Pumpkin seeds and sunflower seeds are rich in zinc, which is important for immune function and hormone balance.
- Chia and flaxseeds are excellent sources of omega-3 fatty acids, which can help reduce inflammation and support brain health.
- The cinnamon and salt (if used) can add flavor without the need for added sugars.

Instructions:

1. In a medium bowl, combine the almonds, walnuts, pumpkin seeds, sunflower seeds, chia seeds, and ground flaxseeds.

2. If desired, sprinkle the cinnamon and sea salt over the nut and seed mixture and stir to combine.

3. Divide the mixed nuts and seeds into 4 individual servings and store in airtight containers or resealable bags.

Tips:
- You can adjust the ratios of nuts and seeds to your personal preference.
- For added crunch, you can lightly toast the nuts and seeds before mixing them together.
- This snack can be enjoyed on its own or added to yogurt, oatmeal, or salads.

Enjoy this nutrient-dense and satisfying snack as part of your menopause-friendly diet.

73. Cherry Tomatoes with Mozzarella Balls

Ingredients:

- 1 pint (about 12 oz) cherry tomatoes, halved
- 8 oz fresh mozzarella balls, halved
- 2 tablespoons balsamic glaze
- 1 tablespoon extra-virgin olive oil
- 2 tablespoons chopped fresh basil
- 1/4 teaspoon sea salt
- 1/4 teaspoon ground black pepper

PreparationTime: 10 minutes
Cook Time: 0 minutes
Total Time: 10 minutes
Serves: 4 servings

Nutritional Benefits for Menopause:
- Cherry tomatoes are a good source of lycopene, an antioxidant that may help reduce the risk of certain health conditions associated with menopause.
- Mozzarella cheese is a lean protein source that can help maintain muscle mass during the menopausal transition.
- The balsamic glaze and olive oil provide healthy fats that can help with hormone balance and overall health.
- Fresh basil is rich in antioxidants and can add flavor without the need for added salt or sugar.

Instructions:

1. In a medium bowl, gently toss the halved cherry tomatoes and mozzarella balls.

2. Drizzle the balsamic glaze and olive oil over the tomato and mozzarella mixture, and then sprinkle with the chopped fresh basil, sea salt, and ground black pepper.

3. Gently toss the ingredients to combine and ensure the tomatoes and mozzarella are evenly coated.

4. Serve immediately or refrigerate until ready to serve.

Tips:
- For a creamier texture, you can use small mozzarella pearls instead of larger mozzarella balls.
- If you prefer a tangier flavor, you can use a balsamic vinegar instead of the balsamic glaze.
- This dish can be served as a light appetizer, side dish, or even a main course when paired with a salad or whole-grain crackers.

Enjoy this refreshing and nutritious snack or side dish during your menopause journey!

74. Baked Sweet Potato Fries

Ingredients:

- 2 medium sweet potatoes, peeled
and cut into 1/2-inch thick fry-shaped pieces
- 1 tablespoon olive oil
- 1 teaspoon paprika
- 1/2 teaspoon garlic powder
- 1/4 teaspoon ground cumin
- 1/4 teaspoon sea salt
- 1/4 teaspoon ground black pepper

Sides and Snacks

PreparationTime: 15 minutes
Cook Time: 25-30 minutes
Total Time: 40-45 minutes
Serves: 4 servings

Nutritional Benefits for Menopause:
- Sweet potatoes are a great source of beta-carotene, which can help support skin and eye health during menopause.
- The complex carbohydrates in sweet potatoes can help regulate blood sugar levels, which is important for managing menopausal symptoms.
- The spices used in this recipe, such as paprika and cumin, are rich in antioxidants that can help reduce inflammation.
- Baking the sweet potato fries instead of frying them helps to reduce the amount of unhealthy fats in the dish.

Instructions:

1. Preheat your oven to 400°F (200°C). Line a baking sheet with parchment paper or a silicone baking mat.

2. Wash and peel the sweet potatoes. Cut them into 1/2-inch thick fry-shaped pieces.

3. In a large bowl, toss the sweet potato fries with the olive oil, paprika, garlic powder, cumin, sea salt, and black pepper until they are evenly coated.

4. Spread the seasoned sweet potato fries in a single layer on the prepared baking sheet.

5. Bake the fries in the preheated oven for 25-30 minutes, flipping them halfway through, until they are crispy and golden brown.

6. Remove the baked sweet potato fries from the oven and serve hot.

Enjoy these nutritious and flavorful baked sweet potato fries as part of your menopause-friendly diet!

75. Kale Chips with Sea Salt

Ingredients:

- 1 bunch of kale, stems removed and
leaves torn into bite-sized pieces (about 4 cups)
- 1 tablespoon olive oil
- 1/4 teaspoon sea salt

PreparationTime: 10 minutes
Cook Time: 12-15 minutes
Total Time: 22-25 minutes
Serves: 4 servings

Nutritional Benefits for Menopause:

- Kale is an excellent source of vitamins A, C, and K, as well as calcium and magnesium, which are important for bone health during menopause.

- The antioxidants in kale, such as lutein and zeaxanthin, can help support eye health and reduce the risk of age-related macular degeneration.

- The healthy fats from the olive oil can help with hormone balance and overall cardiovascular health.
- The sea salt provides a flavorful alternative to processed, high-sodium snacks.

Instructions:

1. Preheat your oven to 350°F (175°C). Line a large baking sheet with parchment paper.

2. Wash the kale leaves and pat them dry thoroughly with a clean kitchen towel or paper towels.

3. In a large bowl, toss the kale leaves with the olive oil until they are evenly coated.

4. Spread the kale leaves in a single layer on the prepared baking sheet, making sure they are not overlapping.

5. Sprinkle the sea salt evenly over the kale leaves.

6. Bake the kale chips in the preheated oven for 12-15 minutes, or until they are crispy and lightly browned.

7. Remove the kale chips from the oven and let them cool for a few minutes before serving.

These crispy and flavorful kale chips are a nutritious and satisfying alternative to traditional snacks, making them a great choice for a menopause-friendly diet.

76. Whole Grain Crackers with Cheese

Ingredients:

- 4-6 whole grain crackers
- 1 ounce (28g) low-fat or
reduced-fat cheddar cheese, sliced or cubed

PreparationTime: 5 minutes
Cook Time: 0 minutes
Total Time: 5 minutes
Serves: 1 serving

Nutritional Benefits for Menopause:

- Whole grain crackers are a good source of complex carbohydrates, fiber, and B vitamins, which can help maintain energy levels and support overall health during menopause.

- Cheddar cheese is a lean protein source that can help maintain muscle mass and support bone health.

- The combination of the whole grains and protein-rich cheese provides a satisfying and nutrient-dense snack.

Instructions:

1. Arrange the whole grain crackers on a plate or small serving board.

2. Top each cracker with a slice or cube of the low-fat or reduced-fat cheddar cheese.

Tips:
- Choose whole grain crackers that are high in fiber and low in added sugars and sodium.
- You can also use other types of cheese, such as goat cheese, feta, or low-fat mozzarella, for variety.
- For extra flavor, you can add a sprinkle of dried herbs, such as oregano or basil, or a drizzle of honey or balsamic glaze.
- This snack can be enjoyed on its own or paired with fresh fruit, such as apple slices or grapes, for a more complete and satisfying treat.

This simple and nutritious snack is a great option for a menopause-friendly diet. The combination of the whole grains, protein, and healthy fats can help keep you feeling full and satisfied between meals.

77. Ants on a Log (Celery with Peanut Butter and Raisins)

Ingredients:

- 2-3 celery stalks, cut into 4-inch pieces
- 2 tablespoons natural,
unsweetened peanut butter
- 2 tablespoons raisins

PreparationTime: 5 minutes
Cook Time: 0 minutes
Total Time: 5 minutes
Serves: 1 serving

Nutritional Benefits for Menopause:
- Celery is a low-calorie, high-fiber vegetable that can help with weight management and digestion during menopause.

- Peanut butter is a good source of protein, which can help maintain muscle mass and support overall health.

- Raisins are a natural source of sweetness and contain antioxidants, as well as minerals like iron and potassium, which can be beneficial during the menopausal transition.

Instructions:

1. Wash the celery stalks and cut them into 4-inch pieces.

2. Spread the peanut butter evenly into the "trough" of each celery stick.

3. Top the peanut butter with a few raisins, creating the "ants on a log" appearance.

Tips:
- Choose a natural, unsweetened peanut butter to avoid added sugars.
- You can also use other nut or seed butters, such as almond butter or sunflower seed butter, for variety.
- For extra flavor, you can sprinkle a pinch of cinnamon or a drizzle of honey on top of the peanut butter.
- This snack can be enjoyed as a quick and easy option or as part of a larger meal.

This classic and nutritious snack is a great choice for a menopause-friendly diet. The combination of the crunchy celery, creamy peanut butter, and sweet raisins provides a satisfying and balanced treat.

78. Hard-Boiled Eggs

Ingredients:

- 16 large eggs

Nutritional Benefits for Menopause:
- Eggs are an excellent source of
 high-quality protein, which can help
maintain muscle mass and support
 overall health during menopause.

PreparationTime: 10 minutes
Cook Time: 12 minutes
Total Time: 22 minutes
Serves: 4 servings (4 eggs per
serving)

- Eggs also contain important nutrients like choline, which is essential for brain health and can help with cognitive function.

- The combination of protein and nutrients in eggs can help with feelings of satiety, which can be beneficial for weight management during the menopausal transition.

Instructions:

1. Place the eggs in a single layer in a large saucepan and cover with cold water by 1 inch.

2. Bring the water to a boil over high heat.

3. Once the water reaches a rolling boil, remove the pan from the heat and cover with a lid.

4. Let the eggs sit in the hot water for 12 minutes for large eggs.

5. Drain the hot water and cover the eggs with cold water to stop the cooking process.

6. Let the eggs sit in the cold water for 5 minutes.

7. Peel the eggs and enjoy them as a snack or incorporate them into other dishes.

Tips:
- Adjust the cooking time based on the size of the eggs (smaller eggs may need less time, larger eggs may need more).
- Hard-boiled eggs can be stored in the refrigerator for up to 1 week, making them a convenient and versatile option for a menopause-friendly diet.
- You can season the hard-boiled eggs with a sprinkle of salt, pepper, or other spices to add flavor.

79. Fresh Veggie Platter with Hummus

Ingredients:

Sides and Snacks

Veggie Platter:
- 1 cup baby carrots
- 1 cup cucumber slices
- 1 cup cherry tomatoes, halved
- 1 cup broccoli florets
- 1 cup cauliflower florets
- 1 cup bell pepper strips (red, yellow, or orange)

PreparationTime: 15 minutes
Cook Time: 0 minutes
Total Time: 15 minutes
Serves: 4-6 servings

Hummus:
- 1 (15 oz) can chickpeas, drained and rinsed
- 2 tablespoons tahini
- 2 tablespoons fresh lemon juice
- 1 garlic clove, minced
- 2 tablespoons olive oil
- 1/4 teaspoon ground cumin
- 1/4 teaspoon sea salt
- 2-3 tablespoons water (as needed)

Nutritional Benefits for Menopause:
- The variety of fresh vegetables provides a range of vitamins, minerals, and antioxidants that can support overall health during menopause.
- Hummus is a good source of plant-based protein, fiber, and healthy fats from the chickpeas and tahini, which can help with satiety and blood sugar regulation.
- The lemon juice and garlic in the hummus provide additional anti-inflammatory benefits.

Instructions:
1. Prepare the veggie platter by arranging the baby carrots, cucumber slices, cherry tomatoes, broccoli florets, cauliflower florets, and bell pepper strips on a large serving plate or board.

Hummus:
1. In a food processor or high-speed blender, combine the drained and rinsed chickpeas, tahini, lemon juice, garlic, olive oil, cumin, and sea salt.
2. Blend the ingredients until smooth, adding 2-3 tablespoons of water as needed to achieve the desired consistency.
3. Transfer the hummus to a serving bowl and place it in the center of the veggie platter.

Serve the fresh veggie platter with the homemade hummus dip. Enjoy this nutritious and satisfying snack or appetizer as part of your menopause-friendly diet.

Tips:
- You can adjust the types of vegetables based on your personal preferences or what's in season.

80. Avocado Slices with Lime and Sea Salt

Ingredients:

- 1 ripe avocado, sliced
- 1 tablespoon fresh lime juice
- 1/4 teaspoon coarse sea salt

Sides and Snacks

PreparationTime: 5 minutes
Cook Time: 0 minutes
Total Time: 5 minutes
Serves: 1 serving

Nutritional Benefits for Menopause:

- Avocados are an excellent source of healthy monounsaturated fats, which can help support hormone balance and cardiovascular health during menopause.

- Avocados are also rich in fiber, vitamins, and minerals, including potassium, which can help with fluid balance and muscle function.

- The lime juice provides a refreshing, tangy flavor and a boost of vitamin C, which is important for immune function and collagen production.

- The sea salt adds a flavorful touch without the need for excessive sodium.

Instructions:

1. Slice the avocado in half, remove the pit, and then slice the avocado flesh into thin, even slices.

2. Arrange the avocado slices on a plate or small serving dish.

3. Drizzle the fresh lime juice evenly over the avocado slices.

4. Sprinkle the coarse sea salt over the avocado slices.

Tips:
- For extra flavor, you can also add a sprinkle of ground black pepper or a pinch of chili powder.
- Serve the avocado slices immediately for the best texture and flavor.
- This simple snack can be enjoyed on its own or paired with whole-grain crackers or a small salad for a more substantial meal.

Enjoy these creamy, tangy, and flavorful avocado slices as a nutritious and satisfying snack during your menopause journey.

81. Baked Apples with Cinnamon

Ingredients:

- 4 medium-sized apples
(such as Gala, Honeycrisp, or Fuji)
- 2 tablespoons unsweetened applesauce
- 1 teaspoon ground cinnamon
- 1/4 teaspoon ground nutmeg (optional)
- 2 tablespoons chopped walnuts or pecans (optional)
- 1 tablespoon honey or maple syrup (optional)

Sweet and Healthy Desserts

PreparationTime: 10 minutes
Cook Time: 30 minutes
Total Time: 40 minutes
Serves: 4 servings

Nutritional Benefits for Menopause:
- Apples are a good source of fiber, which can help with digestion and weight management during menopause.
- Cinnamon is an antioxidant-rich spice that may help regulate blood sugar levels and reduce inflammation.
- Walnuts and pecans provide healthy fats and protein, which can help maintain muscle mass and support overall health.
- The natural sweetness from the apples and optional honey or maple syrup can satisfy cravings without the need for added sugars.

Instructions:
1. Preheat your oven to 375°F (190°C).

2. Wash and core the apples, leaving a small well in the center of each one.

3. In a small bowl, mix together the unsweetened applesauce, cinnamon, and nutmeg (if using).

4. Spoon the cinnamon-applesauce mixture into the center of each apple.

5. If using, sprinkle the chopped walnuts or pecans over the top of the apples.

6. Place the stuffed apples in a baking dish and bake for 30-35 minutes, or until the apples are tender and the filling is bubbly.

7. Remove the baked apples from the oven and drizzle with a small amount of honey or maple syrup, if desired.

8. Serve the baked apples warm, either on their own or with a dollop of plain Greek yogurt or a sprinkle of additional cinnamon.

Tips:
- For a creamier filling, you can mix the applesauce with a small amount of softened cream cheese or mascarpone.
- Experiment with different spice combinations, such as ginger, allspice, or cardamom, to find your favorite flavor profile.

82. Chia Seed Pudding with Mango

Ingredients:

- 1/4 cup chia seeds
- 1 cup unsweetened almond milk
- 1 tablespoon honey (or maple syrup)
- 1/2 teaspoon vanilla extract
- 1 cup diced fresh mango

Sweet and Healthy Desserts

PreparationTime: 10 minutes
Chilling Time: 2-4 hours
Total Time: 2-4 hours 10 minutes
Serves: 4 servings

Nutritional Benefits for Menopause:
- Chia seeds are an excellent source of omega-3 fatty acids, fiber, and protein, which can help support hormone balance and overall health during menopause.
- Mangoes are rich in vitamins A and C, as well as antioxidants, which can help reduce inflammation and support skin health.
- The honey (or maple syrup) provides a natural sweetener without the need for added sugars.
- Almond milk is a dairy-free, low-calorie option that is easy to digest.

Instructions:

1. In a medium bowl, whisk together the chia seeds, almond milk, honey, and vanilla extract until well combined.

2. Cover the bowl and refrigerate for 2-4 hours, or until the chia seeds have thickened the mixture into a pudding-like consistency. Stir the mixture occasionally during this time.

3. Once the chia seed pudding has set, divide it evenly into 4 serving bowls or cups.

4. Top each serving of chia seed pudding with 1/4 cup of diced fresh mango.

5. Serve chilled and enjoy!

Tips:
- For a creamier texture, you can use full-fat coconut milk instead of almond milk.
- Experiment with different fruit toppings, such as berries or kiwi, to vary the flavors.
- You can make the chia seed pudding in advance and store it in the refrigerator for up to 4 days.

This nutrient-dense chia seed pudding with fresh mango is a delicious and satisfying treat that can be enjoyed as a healthy breakfast, snack, or dessert during your menopause journey.

83. Dark Chocolate Covered Almonds

Ingredients:

- 1 cup raw, unsalted almonds
- 2 ounces dark chocolate
(70% cacao or higher), melted

Nutritional Benefits for Menopause:

PreparationTime: 10 minutes
Cook Time: 0 minutes
Total Time: 10 minutes
Serves: 4 servings (about 1/4 cup per serving)

- Almonds are a good source of healthy fats, protein, fiber, and magnesium, which can help support bone health and hormone balance during menopause.
- Dark chocolate is rich in antioxidants and can help reduce inflammation, which is important for overall health during the menopausal transition.
- The combination of the healthy fats from the almonds and the antioxidants from the dark chocolate can provide a satisfying and nutrient-dense snack.

Instructions:

1. Line a baking sheet with parchment paper or a silicone baking mat.

2. In a small bowl, melt the dark chocolate using a double boiler or by microwaving in 30-second intervals, stirring frequently, until smooth.

3. Add the raw, unsalted almonds to the melted chocolate and stir to coat the almonds evenly.

4. Using a spoon or fork, transfer the chocolate-covered almonds to the prepared baking sheet, spreading them out in a single layer.

5. Place the baking sheet in the refrigerator and chill for at least 30 minutes, or until the chocolate has hardened.

6. Once the chocolate has set, break apart any almonds that have stuck together and transfer the dark chocolate-covered almonds to an airtight container. Store the chocolate-covered almonds in the refrigerator for up to 1 week.

Tips:
- For extra flavor, you can add a pinch of sea salt or a sprinkle of cinnamon to the melted chocolate before coating the almonds.
- You can also experiment with different types of nuts, such as cashews or hazelnuts, for variety.
- Portion the chocolate-covered almonds into individual servings to help with portion control.

84. Frozen Yogurt Bark with Berries

Ingredients:

- 2 cups plain Greek yogurt
- 2 tablespoons honey (or maple syrup)
- 1 teaspoon vanilla extract
- 1 cup mixed berries
 (such as blueberries, raspberries, and blackberries)
- 2 tablespoons chopped walnuts or almonds (optional)

Sweet and Healthy Desserts

PreparationTime: 15 minutes
Freezing Time: 2-3 hours
Total Time: 2-3 hours 15 minutes
Serves: 6 servings

Nutritional Benefits for Menopause:
- Greek yogurt is a good source of protein, which can help maintain muscle mass during menopause.
- Berries are rich in antioxidants, fiber, and vitamins that can support overall health and reduce inflammation.
- Walnuts and almonds provide healthy fats and additional protein, which can help with feelings of satiety.
- The honey (or maple syrup) adds natural sweetness without the need for added sugars.

Instructions:

1. Line a baking sheet with parchment paper or a silicone baking mat.

2. In a medium bowl, mix together the Greek yogurt, honey (or maple syrup), and vanilla extract until well combined.

3. Spread the yogurt mixture evenly onto the prepared baking sheet, creating a thin, even layer.

4. Sprinkle the mixed berries and chopped nuts (if using) over the top of the yogurt layer.

5. Place the baking sheet in the freezer and freeze for 2-3 hours, or until the yogurt bark is completely frozen.

6. Once frozen, break the yogurt bark into pieces and transfer to an airtight container or resealable bag. Store the frozen yogurt bark in the freezer for up to 2 months.

Tips:
- You can use any combination of fresh or frozen berries that you prefer.
- For a creamier texture, you can use full-fat Greek yogurt instead of low-fat.
- Experiment with different toppings, such as shredded coconut, chia seeds, or a drizzle of melted dark chocolate.
- Enjoy the frozen yogurt bark as a healthy snack or dessert during your menopause journey.

This refreshing and nutrient-dense frozen yogurt bark is a great way to satisfy your sweet tooth while supporting your overall health during menopause.

85. Banana Ice Cream with Peanut Butter Swirl

Ingredients:

- 4 ripe bananas, peeled and sliced
- 2 tablespoons natural, unsweetened peanut butter
- 1 tablespoon honey (optional)

Nutritional Benefits for Menopause:

Sweet and Healthy Desserts

PreparationTime: 10 minutes
Freezing Time: 4-6 hours
Total Time: 4-6 hours 10 minutes
Serves: 4 servings

- Bananas are a good source of potassium, which can help with muscle function and bone health during menopause.
- Peanut butter provides healthy fats and protein, which can help maintain muscle mass and support overall health.
- The honey (if used) adds a natural sweetener without the need for added sugars.

Instructions:

1. In a single layer, arrange the sliced bananas on a baking sheet or plate. Place the baking sheet or plate in the freezer and freeze for at least 4-6 hours, or until the bananas are completely frozen.

2. Once the bananas are frozen, transfer them to a high-speed blender or food processor.

3. Blend the frozen bananas until they reach a smooth, creamy, and ice cream-like consistency, scraping down the sides as needed.

4. In a small microwave-safe bowl, heat the peanut butter for 20-30 seconds, or until it's slightly softened and drizzle-able.

5. Scoop the banana "ice cream" into serving bowls or cups. Drizzle the warmed peanut butter over the top of the banana ice cream, creating a swirl pattern.

6. If desired, drizzle a small amount of honey over the peanut butter swirl. Serve immediately and enjoy the frozen treat.

Tips:
- For a creamier texture, you can add a splash of unsweetened almond milk or coconut milk to the blended bananas.
- Experiment with different nut butters, such as almond butter or cashew butter, for variety.
- You can also add a sprinkle of cinnamon or a pinch of sea salt to the banana ice cream for extra flavor.
- This recipe can be easily doubled or tripled to make a larger batch.

This simple and nutritious banana ice cream with a peanut butter swirl is a delicious and satisfying treat that can be enjoyed during your menopause journey.

86. Oatmeal Raisin Cookies

Ingredients:

- 1 cup whole wheat flour
- 1 teaspoon baking soda
- 1/2 teaspoon ground cinnamon
- 1/4 teaspoon ground nutmeg
- 1/4 teaspoon salt
- 1/2 cup unsalted butter, softened
- 1/2 cup brown sugar
- 1 large egg
- 1 teaspoon vanilla extract
- 1 1/2 cups old-fashioned oats
- 3/4 cup raisins

Instructions:

1. Preheat your oven to 350°F (175°C). Line a baking sheet with parchment paper.

2. In a medium bowl, whisk together the whole wheat flour, baking soda, cinnamon, nutmeg, and salt.

3. In a large bowl, cream the softened butter and brown sugar together until light and fluffy.

4. Beat in the egg and vanilla extract until well combined.

5. Gradually stir the dry ingredients into the wet ingredients until just combined.

6. Fold in the old-fashioned oats and raisins.

7. Scoop rounded tablespoons of the dough onto the prepared baking sheet, spacing them about 2 inches apart.

8. Bake the cookies for 12-15 minutes, or until they are lightly golden brown.

9. Remove the cookies from the oven and let them cool on the baking sheet for 5 minutes before transferring them to a wire rack to cool completely.

Tips:
- For a chewier texture, bake the cookies for the shorter end of the time range.
- You can also add chopped walnuts or pecans for extra crunch and healthy fats.
- Store the cooled cookies in an airtight container at room temperature for up to 1 week.

Enjoy these wholesome and delicious oatmeal raisin cookies as a satisfying treat during your menopause journey.

PreparationTime: 15 minutes
Baking Time: 12-15 minutes
Total Time: 27-30 minutes
Serves: 18 cookies

87. Blueberry Greek Yogurt Parfait

Ingredients:

- 1 cup plain Greek yogurt
- 1/2 cup fresh or frozen blueberries
- 2 tablespoons chopped walnuts
- 1 tablespoon honey (optional)

PreparationTime: 10 minutes
Total Time: 10 minutes
Serves: 2 servings

Nutritional Benefits for Menopause:
- Greek yogurt is a good source of protein, which can help maintain muscle mass during menopause.
- Blueberries are rich in antioxidants, fiber, and vitamins that can support overall health and reduce inflammation.
- Walnuts provide healthy fats and additional protein, which can help with feelings of satiety.
- The honey (if used) adds natural sweetness without the need for added sugars.

Instructions:

1. In a small glass or jar, layer half of the Greek yogurt.

2. Top the yogurt with half of the blueberries.

3. Sprinkle half of the chopped walnuts over the blueberries.

4. Repeat the layers, ending with the remaining yogurt, blueberries, and walnuts.

5. If desired, drizzle the honey over the top of the parfait.

6. Serve immediately or refrigerate until ready to enjoy.

Tips:
- You can use any type of fresh or frozen berries, such as raspberries or blackberries, in place of the blueberries.
- For a creamier texture, you can use full-fat Greek yogurt instead of low-fat.
- Experiment with different toppings, such as granola, chia seeds, or a sprinkle of cinnamon.
- This parfait can be made in advance and stored in the refrigerator for up to 3 days.

This refreshing and nutrient-dense Blueberry Greek Yogurt Parfait is a great option for a healthy breakfast, snack, or dessert during your menopause journey.

88. Almond Flour Brownies

Ingredients:

- 1 cup almond flour
- 1/4 cup unsweetened cocoa powder
- 1/4 teaspoon baking soda
- 1/4 teaspoon salt
- 1/2 cup unsalted butter, melted
- 3/4 cup granulated erythritol or monk fruit sweetener
- 2 large eggs
- 1 teaspoon vanilla extract
- 1/4 cup chopped walnuts or pecans (optional)

PreparationTime: 15 minutes
Baking Time: 20-25 minutes
Total Time: 35-40 minutes
Serves: 16 brownies

Nutritional Benefits for Menopause:
- Almond flour is a low-carb, high-fiber, and protein-rich alternative to traditional flour, which can help manage blood sugar levels during menopause.
- Cocoa powder is a good source of antioxidants that can help reduce inflammation.
- Walnuts and pecans provide healthy fats and additional protein, which can help maintain muscle mass.
- Erythritol and monk fruit sweetener are low-calorie, natural sweeteners that do not spike blood sugar levels.

Instructions:
1. Preheat your oven to 350°F (175°C). Grease an 8x8-inch baking pan with non-stick cooking spray or line it with parchment paper.

2. In a medium bowl, whisk together the almond flour, cocoa powder, baking soda, and salt.

3. In a separate bowl, whisk together the melted butter, erythritol (or monk fruit sweetener), eggs, and vanilla extract until well combined.

4. Gradually stir the wet ingredients into the dry ingredients until just combined. Do not overmix.

5. If using, fold in the chopped walnuts or pecans.

6. Spread the brownie batter evenly into the prepared baking pan.

7. Bake for 20-25 minutes, or until a toothpick inserted into the center comes out clean.

8. Allow the brownies to cool completely in the pan before cutting into 16 squares.

Tips:
- For a fudgier texture, bake the brownies for the shorter end of the time range.
- You can also add a sprinkle of sea salt on top of the brownies for a sweet and salty contrast.
- Store the cooled brownies in an airtight container at room temperature for up to 5 days.

89. Coconut Macaroons

Ingredients:

- 2 cups unsweetened shredded coconut
- 1/4 cup granulated erythritol or monk fruit sweetener
- 2 large egg whites
- 1/4 teaspoon vanilla extract
- 1/8 teaspoon salt

PreparationTime: 10 minutes
Baking Time: 12-15 minutes
Total Time: 22-25 minutes
Serves: 12 macaroons

Nutritional Benefits for Menopause:
- Coconut is a good source of healthy fats, which can help support hormone balance and brain health during menopause.
- Egg whites provide a lean source of protein to help maintain muscle mass.
- Erythritol and monk fruit sweetener are low-calorie, natural sweeteners that do not spike blood sugar levels.

Instructions:

1. Preheat your oven to 325°F (165°C). Line a baking sheet with parchment paper.

2. In a medium bowl, mix together the unsweetened shredded coconut and the granulated erythritol (or monk fruit sweetener).

3. In a separate small bowl, beat the egg whites until they are foamy and hold soft peaks.

4. Gently fold the beaten egg whites and vanilla extract into the coconut mixture until well combined.

5. Scoop rounded tablespoons of the coconut mixture and place them about 1 inch apart on the prepared baking sheet.

6. Bake the macaroons for 12-15 minutes, or until they are lightly golden brown on the edges.

7. Remove the macaroons from the oven and let them cool on the baking sheet for 5 minutes before transferring them to a wire rack to cool completely.

Tips:
- For a chewier texture, bake the macaroons for the shorter end of the time range.
- You can also add a small amount of unsweetened shredded coconut on top of the macaroons before baking for extra coconut flavor.
- Store the cooled macaroons in an airtight container at room temperature for up to 1 week.

These delicious and nutritious Coconut Macaroons are a great option for a menopause-friendly treat or snack.

90. Pumpkin Muffins with Almond Flour

Ingredients:

- 1 1/2 cups almond flour
- 1 teaspoon baking soda
- 1 teaspoon ground cinnamon
- 1/2 teaspoon ground ginger
- 1/4 teaspoon ground nutmeg
- 1/4 teaspoon salt
- 3 large eggs
- 1/2 cup unsweetened pumpkin puree
- 1/4 cup granulated erythritol or monk fruit sweetener
- 2 tablespoons melted coconut oil
- 1 teaspoon vanilla extract

Sweet and Healthy Desserts

PreparationTime: 15 minutes
Baking Time: 20-25 minutes
Total Time: 35-40 minutes
Serves: 12 muffins

Nutritional Benefits for Menopause:
- Almond flour is a low-carb, high-fiber, and protein-rich alternative to traditional flour, which can help manage blood sugar levels during menopause.
- Pumpkin is a good source of beta-carotene, which can support skin and eye health.
- The spices, such as cinnamon and ginger, are rich in antioxidants that can help reduce inflammation.
- Erythritol and monk fruit sweetener are low-calorie, natural sweeteners that do not spike blood sugar levels.

Instructions:

1. Preheat your oven to 350°F (175°C). Grease a 12-cup muffin tin or line it with paper liners.

2. In a medium bowl, whisk together the almond flour, baking soda, cinnamon, ginger, nutmeg, and salt.

3. In a separate large bowl, beat the eggs. Then, stir in the pumpkin puree, erythritol (or monk fruit sweetener), melted coconut oil, and vanilla extract until well combined.

4. Gradually fold the dry ingredients into the wet ingredients, mixing just until combined. Do not overmix.

5. Divide the batter evenly among the prepared muffin cups, filling them about 3/4 full.

6. Bake the muffins for 20-25 minutes, or until a toothpick inserted into the center comes out clean.

7. Allow the muffins to cool in the tin for 5 minutes before transferring them to a wire rack to cool completely.

91. Fruit Sorbet with Fresh Mint

Ingredients:

- 2 cups pureed fruit
 (such as mango, pineapple, or berries)
- 1 cup water
- 3/4 cup sugar
- 2 tablespoons fresh lemon juice
- 1/4 cup chopped fresh mint leaves

PreparationTime: 10 minutes
Cook Time: 5 minutes
Total Time: 2 hours 15 minutes
Serves: 4-6

Instructions:

1. In a medium saucepan, combine the pureed fruit, water, and sugar. Bring to a simmer over medium heat, stirring occasionally, until the sugar has dissolved, about 5 minutes. Remove from heat and stir in the lemon juice.

2. Pour the mixture into a shallow baking dish and place in the freezer. Stir the mixture every 30 minutes with a fork to break up any ice crystals that form, until it reaches a sorbet-like consistency, about 2-3 hours.

3. Once the sorbet is frozen, transfer it to a food processor or blender. Add the chopped fresh mint and pulse until the mint is finely chopped and incorporated throughout the sorbet.

4. Return the sorbet to the freezer and freeze for an additional 1-2 hours, stirring occasionally, until firm.

5. Scoop the sorbet into bowls or glasses and serve immediately, garnished with additional fresh mint if desired.

Enjoy your refreshing and flavorful Fruit Sorbet with Fresh Mint!

92. Dark Chocolate and Raspberry Squares

Ingredients:

- 1 cup unsweetened cocoa powder
- 1/2 cup coconut flour
- 1/4 cup ground flaxseed
- 1/4 cup erythritol or other low-calorie sweetener
- 1/4 teaspoon sea salt
- 1/2 cup coconut oil, melted
- 1/4 cup unsweetened almond milk
- 1 teaspoon vanilla extract
- 1 cup fresh or frozen raspberries

PreparationTime: 15 minutes
Cook Time: 20 minutes
Total Time: 35 minutes
Serves: 16 squares

Instructions:

1. Preheat the oven to 350°F (175°C). Line an 8x8-inch baking pan with parchment paper.

2. In a medium bowl, whisk together the cocoa powder, coconut flour, ground flaxseed, erythritol, and sea salt.

3. In a separate bowl, combine the melted coconut oil, almond milk, and vanilla extract.

4. Pour the wet ingredients into the dry ingredients and mix until well combined.

5. Gently fold in the raspberries, being careful not to crush them.

6. Spread the mixture evenly into the prepared baking pan.

7. Bake for 18-20 minutes, or until the edges are set and the center is still slightly soft.

8. Allow the squares to cool completely in the pan before cutting into 16 pieces.

9. Store the squares in an airtight container in the refrigerator for up to 1 week.

These Dark Chocolate and Raspberry Squares are a delicious and healthy treat for those following a menopause diet. The combination of dark chocolate, raspberries, and low-calorie ingredients makes them a great source of antioxidants and fiber, while also being low in sugar and carbohydrates.

93. Lemon Chia Seed Muffins

Ingredients:

- 1 1/2 cups whole wheat flour
- 1/2 cup ground flaxseed
- 1/4 cup chia seeds
- 1 teaspoon baking powder
- 1/2 teaspoon baking soda
- 1/4 teaspoon salt
- 1/2 cup unsweetened applesauce
- 1/2 cup honey
- 1/4 cup unsweetened almond milk
- 2 tablespoons lemon juice
- 1 tablespoon lemon zest

Sweet and Healthy Desserts

PreparationTime: 15 minutes
Cook Time: 20 minutes
Total Time: 35 minutes
Serves: 12 muffins

Instructions:

1. Preheat the oven to 375°F (190°C). Grease a 12-cup muffin tin or line with paper liners.

2. In a large bowl, whisk together the whole wheat flour, ground flaxseed, chia seeds, baking powder, baking soda, and salt.

3. In a separate bowl, combine the unsweetened applesauce, honey, almond milk, lemon juice, and lemon zest.

4. Pour the wet ingredients into the dry ingredients and stir just until combined, being careful not to overmix.

5. Divide the batter evenly among the prepared muffin cups, filling them about 3/4 full.

6. Bake for 18-20 minutes, or until a toothpick inserted into the center comes out clean.

7. Allow the muffins to cool in the tin for 5 minutes before transferring to a wire rack to cool completely.

These Lemon Chia Seed Muffins are a delicious and nutritious breakfast or snack option. The combination of whole wheat flour, flaxseed, and chia seeds provides a good source of fiber, while the lemon flavor and honey add a touch of sweetness without too much sugar.

94. Pear and Almond Tart

Ingredients:

- 1 1/2 cups almond flour
- 1/4 cup coconut flour
- 2 tablespoons ground flaxseed
- 1/4 teaspoon sea salt
- 3 tablespoons coconut oil, melted
- 2 tablespoons honey

Filling Ingredients:
- 3 medium pears, peeled, cored, and thinly sliced
- 1/4 cup unsweetened almond milk
- 2 tablespoons honey
- 1 teaspoon vanilla extract
- 1/4 teaspoon ground cinnamon
- 1/4 cup sliced almonds

PreparationTime: 20 minutes
Cook Time: 40 minutes
Total Time: 1 hour
Serves: 8-10 slices

Crust

Instructions:
1. Preheat the oven to 350°F (175°C). Grease a 9-inch tart pan with a removable bottom.

2. In a medium bowl, whisk together the almond flour, coconut flour, ground flaxseed, and sea salt. Add the melted coconut oil and honey, and mix until a dough forms.

3. Press the dough evenly into the bottom and up the sides of the prepared tart pan.

4. In a separate bowl, combine the sliced pears, almond milk, honey, vanilla, and cinnamon. Toss to coat the pears.

5. Arrange the pear slices in a circular pattern on top of the tart crust. Sprinkle the sliced almonds over the top.

6. Bake for 35-40 minutes, or until the crust is golden brown and the pears are tender.

7. Allow the tart to cool completely before removing the outer ring of the tart pan.

8. Serve the Pear and Almond Tart at room temperature or chilled.

This Pear and Almond Tart is a delicious and nutritious dessert option for those following a menopause diet. The almond and coconut flour crust, along with the pears and almonds, provide a good source of healthy fats, fiber, and antioxidants.

95. Strawberry Banana Smoothie Popsicles

Ingredients:

- 1 cup fresh or frozen strawberries
- 1 ripe banana, peeled
- 1/2 cup unsweetened almond milk
- 2 tablespoons plain Greek yogurt
- 1 tablespoon honey (optional)
- 1/2 teaspoon vanilla extract

PreparationTime: 10 minutes
Freeze Time: 4-6 hours
Total Time: 4-6 hours 10 minutes
Serves: 8 popsicles

Instructions:

1. In a blender, combine the strawberries, banana, almond milk, Greek yogurt, honey (if using), and vanilla extract. Blend until smooth and creamy.

2. Carefully pour the smoothie mixture into popsicle molds, leaving a small amount of space at the top for expansion.

3. Insert popsicle sticks into the molds and place in the freezer for 4-6 hours, or until completely frozen.

4. Once frozen, remove the popsicles from the molds and enjoy immediately or store in an airtight container in the freezer for up to 2 months.

These Strawberry Banana Smoothie Popsicles are a refreshing and healthy treat for a menopause diet. The combination of strawberries, banana, and Greek yogurt provides a good source of fiber, vitamins, and protein, while the almond milk and honey (if used) add a touch of sweetness without too much sugar.

The popsicles are a great way to incorporate more fruits and dairy into your diet, and the frozen format can be a refreshing and satisfying snack or dessert during the warmer months.

96. Apricot and Almond Energy Balls

Ingredients:

- 1 cup dried apricots, chopped
- 1 cup raw almonds
- 1/4 cup unsweetened shredded coconut
- 2 tablespoons ground flaxseed
- 1 tablespoon honey
- 1 teaspoon vanilla extract
- 1/4 teaspoon ground cinnamon

Sweet and Healthy Desserts

PreparationTime: 15 minutes
Total Time: 15 minutes
Serves: 12 energy balls

Instructions:

1. In a food processor, pulse the dried apricots and raw almonds until they are finely chopped and start to form a paste.

2. Add the unsweetened shredded coconut, ground flaxseed, honey, vanilla extract, and ground cinnamon. Pulse until the mixture is well combined and starts to stick together.

3. Scoop the mixture by the tablespoonful and roll into small balls, about 1-inch in diameter.

4. Place the energy balls on a parchment-lined baking sheet and refrigerate for at least 30 minutes to allow them to firm up.

5. Store the Apricot and Almond Energy Balls in an airtight container in the refrigerator for up to 1 week.

These Apricot and Almond Energy Balls are a great snack option for a menopause diet. The combination of dried apricots, almonds, and flaxseed provides a good source of fiber, healthy fats, and antioxidants. The honey adds a touch of sweetness without too much sugar.

These energy balls are perfect for a quick and nutritious pick-me-up, and they can also be enjoyed as a healthy dessert or snack. They are easy to make and can be stored in the refrigerator for a convenient and satisfying treat.

97. Mixed Berry Crumble

Ingredients:

- 3 cups mixed berries
- 2 tablespoons honey
- 1 tablespoon arrowroot powder
- 1 teaspoon vanilla extract
- 1/4 teaspoon ground cinnamon

Crumble Topping Ingredients:
- 1 cup almond flour
- 1/2 cup rolled oats
- 1/4 cup chopped pecans
- 2 tablespoons coconut oil, melted
- 2 tablespoons honey
- 1/4 teaspoon sea salt

Sweet and Healthy Desserts

PreparationTime: 20 minutes
Cook Time: 30 minutes
Total Time: 50 minutes
Serves: 6-8

Filling

Instructions:

1. Preheat the oven to 375°F (190°C). Grease an 8x8-inch baking dish.

2. In a large bowl, gently toss together the mixed berries, honey, arrowroot powder, vanilla extract, and cinnamon until well combined.

3. In a separate bowl, mix together the almond flour, rolled oats, chopped pecans, melted coconut oil, honey, and sea salt until the mixture resembles coarse crumbs.

4. Spread the berry mixture evenly into the prepared baking dish. Sprinkle the crumble topping over the top.

5. Bake for 25-30 minutes, or until the topping is golden brown and the berries are bubbling.

6. Allow the crumble to cool for at least 15 minutes before serving.

7. Serve the Mixed Berry Crumble warm, with a scoop of vanilla Greek yogurt or a drizzle of unsweetened almond milk, if desired.

This Mixed Berry Crumble is a delicious and nutritious dessert option for those following a menopause diet. The combination of antioxidant-rich berries, fiber-rich oats and nuts, and healthy fats from the almond flour and coconut oil make this a satisfying and nourishing treat.

98. Honey Roasted Almonds

Ingredients:

- 2 cups raw almonds
- 2 tablespoons honey
- 1 teaspoon ground cinnamon
- 1/4 teaspoon sea salt

PreparationTime: 5 minutes
Cook Time: 15 minutes
Total Time: 20 minutes
Serves: 8 (1/4 cup servings)

Instructions:

1. Preheat the oven to 325°F (165°C). Line a baking sheet with parchment paper.

2. In a medium bowl, toss the raw almonds with the honey, cinnamon, and sea salt until the almonds are evenly coated.

3. Spread the honey-coated almonds in a single layer on the prepared baking sheet.

4. Roast the almonds for 12-15 minutes, stirring halfway, until they are lightly golden and fragrant.

5. Remove the almonds from the oven and let them cool completely on the baking sheet, about 10 minutes.

6. Once cooled, transfer the honey roasted almonds to an airtight container for storage.

These Honey Roasted Almonds make a delicious and nutritious snack for a menopause diet. Almonds are a great source of healthy fats, fiber, and protein, while the honey provides a touch of natural sweetness without added sugar.

The cinnamon adds a warm, comforting flavor and may also help to regulate blood sugar levels. These roasted almonds are perfect for satisfying cravings, providing a quick energy boost, or enjoying as a healthy dessert.

Store the Honey Roasted Almonds in an airtight container at room temperature for up to 2 weeks.

99. Vegan Chocolate Avocado Mousse

Ingredients:

- 2 ripe avocados, pitted and peeled
- 1/2 cup unsweetened cocoa powder
- 1/4 cup maple syrup
- 1/4 cup unsweetened almond milk
- 1 teaspoon vanilla extract
- 1/4 teaspoon sea salt

PreparationTime: 10 minutes
Chilling Time: 2 hours
Total Time: 2 hours 10 minutes
Serves: 4

Instructions:

1. In a food processor or high-speed blender, combine the avocados, cocoa powder, maple syrup, almond milk, vanilla extract, and sea salt. Blend until the mixture is smooth and creamy, scraping down the sides as needed.

2. Divide the chocolate avocado mousse evenly into 4 small ramekins or serving dishes.

3. Cover the mousse and refrigerate for at least 2 hours, or until chilled and set.

4. Serve the Vegan Chocolate Avocado Mousse chilled, garnished with fresh berries, chopped nuts, or a sprinkle of cocoa powder, if desired.

This Vegan Chocolate Avocado Mousse is a delicious and nutritious dessert option for a menopause diet. The avocado provides a creamy, rich texture, while the cocoa powder and maple syrup offer a decadent chocolate flavor without the use of dairy or refined sugar.

Avocados are a great source of healthy fats, fiber, and antioxidants, which can be beneficial during menopause. The almond milk and nuts (if used as a garnish) also contribute to the overall nutrient profile of this dessert.

This mousse is easy to prepare and can be made in advance, making it a convenient and satisfying treat for those following a menopause-friendly diet.

100. Apple and Walnut Crisp

Ingredients:

- 4 cups peeled, cored,
and sliced apples (about 4-5 medium apples)
- 2 tablespoons honey
- 1 tablespoon arrowroot powder
- 1 teaspoon ground cinnamon
- 1/4 teaspoon ground nutmeg

Topping Ingredients:
- 1 cup rolled oats
- 1/2 cup chopped walnuts
- 1/4 cup almond flour
- 2 tablespoons coconut oil, melted
- 2 tablespoons honey
- 1/4 teaspoon sea salt

Sweet and Healthy Desserts

PreparationTime: 20 minutes
Cook Time: 30 minutes
Total Time: 50 minutes
Serves: 6-8

Filling

Instructions:
1. Preheat the oven to 375°F (190°C). Grease an 8x8-inch baking dish.

2. In a large bowl, toss the sliced apples with the honey, arrowroot powder, cinnamon, and nutmeg until the apples are evenly coated. Transfer the apple mixture to the prepared baking dish.

3. In a separate bowl, combine the rolled oats, chopped walnuts, almond flour, melted coconut oil, honey, and sea salt. Mix until the topping is well combined and crumbly.

4. Sprinkle the oat-walnut topping evenly over the apple filling.

5. Bake for 25-30 minutes, or until the topping is golden brown and the apples are tender.

6. Allow the crisp to cool for at least 15 minutes before serving. Serve the Apple and Walnut Crisp warm, with a scoop of vanilla Greek yogurt or a drizzle of unsweetened almond milk, if desired.

This Apple and Walnut Crisp is a delicious and nutritious dessert option for those following a menopause diet. The combination of fiber-rich apples, healthy fats from the walnuts and coconut oil, and natural sweeteners make this a satisfying and nourishing treat. The oats and almond flour in the topping provide additional fiber and nutrients, while the cinnamon and nutmeg add warmth and flavor.

101. Cinnamon Spiced Quinoa Pudding

Ingredients:

- 1 cup uncooked quinoa, rinsed
- 2 cups unsweetened almond milk
- 2 tablespoons honey
- 1 teaspoon ground cinnamon
- 1/4 teaspoon ground nutmeg
- 1/4 teaspoon sea salt
- 1 teaspoon vanilla extract
- 1/4 cup chopped walnuts (optional)

PreparationTime: 10 minutes
Cook Time: 25 minutes
Total Time: 35 minutes
Serves: 4

Instructions:

1. In a medium saucepan, combine the rinsed quinoa and almond milk. Bring the mixture to a boil over medium-high heat.

2. Once boiling, reduce the heat to low, cover the saucepan, and simmer for 15-20 minutes, or until the quinoa is tender and has absorbed most of the liquid.

3. Remove the saucepan from the heat and stir in the honey, cinnamon, nutmeg, sea salt, and vanilla extract. Mix well until the honey is fully incorporated.

4. Allow the quinoa pudding to cool slightly, then transfer it to individual serving bowls or ramekins.

5. Refrigerate the quinoa pudding for at least 30 minutes to allow it to thicken and set.

6. Serve the Cinnamon Spiced Quinoa Pudding chilled, garnished with chopped walnuts (if using).

This Cinnamon Spiced Quinoa Pudding is a delicious and nutritious dessert or snack option for a menopause diet. Quinoa is a gluten-free, high-protein grain that provides fiber, minerals, and antioxidants. The almond milk, honey, and spices add flavor and sweetness without the use of refined sugar.

The walnuts, if included, provide a crunchy texture and additional healthy fats, which can be beneficial during menopause. This pudding is easy to prepare and can be made in advance, making it a convenient and satisfying treat.

102. Mango Coconut Chia Pudding

Ingredients:

- 1 cup unsweetened coconut milk
- 1/4 cup chia seeds
- 2 tablespoons honey
- 1 teaspoon vanilla extract
- 1/4 teaspoon ground cinnamon
- 1 cup diced fresh mango
- 2 tablespoons unsweetened shredded coconut (for topping)

Sweet and Healthy Desserts

PreparationTime: 10 minutes
Chilling Time: 4 hours
Total Time: 4 hours 10 minutes
Serves: 4

Instructions:

1. In a medium bowl, whisk together the coconut milk, chia seeds, honey, vanilla extract, and ground cinnamon until well combined.

2. Cover the bowl and refrigerate for at least 4 hours, or overnight, stirring occasionally, until the chia seeds have thickened the mixture into a pudding-like consistency.

3. Once the chia pudding has set, divide it evenly into 4 serving bowls or jars.

4. Top each serving with 1/4 cup of diced fresh mango and 1/2 tablespoon of unsweetened shredded coconut.

5. Serve chilled and enjoy!

This Mango Coconut Chia Pudding is a delicious and nutritious dessert or snack option for a menopause diet. The chia seeds provide a good source of fiber, protein, and omega-3 fatty acids, while the coconut milk and mango add healthy fats, vitamins, and natural sweetness.

The cinnamon in this recipe may also help to regulate blood sugar levels, which can be beneficial during menopause. This pudding is easy to prepare in advance and can be stored in the refrigerator for up to 4 days, making it a convenient and satisfying treat.

103. Gluten-Free Chocolate Chip Cookies

Ingredients:

- 1 1/4 cups almond flour
- 1/4 cup coconut flour
- 1/2 teaspoon baking soda
- 1/4 teaspoon sea salt
- 1/2 cup coconut oil, melted
- 1/4 cup honey
- 1 egg
- 1 teaspoon vanilla extract
- 1/2 cup dark chocolate chips or chunks

PreparationTime: 15 minutes
Bake Time: 12 minutes
Total Time: 27 minutes
Yields: 18 cookies

Instructions:

1. Preheat the oven to 350°F (175°C). Line a baking sheet with parchment paper.

2. In a medium bowl, whisk together the almond flour, coconut flour, baking soda, and sea salt.

3. In a separate bowl, combine the melted coconut oil, honey, egg, and vanilla extract. Mix until well blended.

4. Pour the wet ingredients into the dry ingredients and stir until just combined. Fold in the dark chocolate chips.

5. Scoop the dough by the tablespoonful and place the cookies about 2 inches apart on the prepared baking sheet.

6. Bake for 10-12 minutes, or until the edges are lightly golden. Be careful not to overbake. Allow the cookies to cool on the baking sheet for 5 minutes before transferring them to a wire rack to cool completely.

These Gluten-Free Chocolate Chip Cookies are a delicious and nutritious treat for a menopause diet. The almond and coconut flours provide a good source of healthy fats and fiber, while the honey adds natural sweetness without refined sugar.

The dark chocolate chips offer antioxidants and a rich chocolate flavor. These cookies are a great option for satisfying cravings or enjoying as a snack. Store them in an airtight container at room temperature for up to 5 days.

104. Almond Butter and Chocolate Energy Bites

Ingredients:

- 1 cup unsweetened almond butter
- 1/4 cup cocoa powder
- 1/4 cup ground flaxseed
- 2 tablespoons honey
- 1 tablespoon chia seeds
- 1/4 teaspoon sea salt

PreparationTime: 10 minutes
Total Time: 10 minutes
Serves: 12 bites

Instructions:

1. In a medium bowl, combine the almond butter, cocoa powder, ground flaxseed, honey, chia seeds, and sea salt. Mix until the ingredients are well incorporated and a sticky dough forms.

2. Using a tablespoon or small cookie scoop, portion the dough into 12 equal-sized balls.

3. Roll each ball between your palms to form a smooth, round energy bite.

4. Place the energy bites on a parchment-lined plate or baking sheet.

5. Refrigerate the bites for at least 30 minutes to allow them to firm up.

6. Serve chilled and enjoy as a quick, nutritious snack.

These Almond Butter and Chocolate Energy Bites are a great option for a menopause diet. The almond butter provides healthy fats and protein, while the cocoa powder and honey offer a touch of sweetness without added refined sugar.

The ground flaxseed and chia seeds are excellent sources of fiber, omega-3 fatty acids, and other essential nutrients that can be beneficial during menopause.

These energy bites are easy to make, portable, and can be stored in the refrigerator for up to 1 week, making them a convenient and satisfying snack option.

105. Zucchini Bread with Walnuts

Ingredients:

- 1 1/2 cups whole wheat flour
- 1/2 cup almond flour
- 1 teaspoon baking soda
- 1/2 teaspoon ground cinnamon
- 1/4 teaspoon ground nutmeg
- 1/4 teaspoon sea salt
- 2 large eggs
- 1/2 cup honey
- 1/3 cup unsweetened applesauce
- 1 teaspoon vanilla extract
- 1 1/2 cups grated zucchini (about 1 medium zucchini)
- 1/2 cup chopped walnuts

PreparationTime: 15 minutes
Bake Time: 55-60 minutes
Total Time: 1 hour 10 minutes
Yields: 1 loaf (12 slices)

Instructions:

1. Preheat the oven to 350°F (175°C). Grease a 9x5-inch loaf pan with non-stick cooking spray or line it with parchment paper.

2. In a medium bowl, whisk together the whole wheat flour, almond flour, baking soda, cinnamon, nutmeg, and sea salt.

3. In a separate large bowl, beat the eggs. Then, stir in the honey, applesauce, and vanilla extract until well combined.

4. Fold the dry ingredients into the wet ingredients until just combined. Gently fold in the grated zucchini and chopped walnuts.

5. Pour the batter into the prepared loaf pan and smooth the top.

6. Bake for 55-60 minutes, or until a toothpick inserted into the center comes out clean.

7. Allow the zucchini bread to cool in the pan for 10 minutes, then transfer it to a wire rack to cool completely before slicing.

This Zucchini Bread with Walnuts is a delicious and nutritious option for a menopause diet. The whole wheat and almond flours provide a good source of fiber, while the zucchini and walnuts add moisture, healthy fats, and beneficial nutrients.

The honey is used as a natural sweetener, and the cinnamon and nutmeg add warmth and flavor without the need for refined sugar.

Enjoy this moist and flavorful zucchini bread as a snack, breakfast, or dessert. It can be stored in an airtight container at room temperature for up to 4 days or in the refrigerator for up to 1 week.

106. Pear and Blueberry Crisp

Ingredients:

- 3 cups diced pears (about 3 medium pears)
- 2 cups fresh or frozen blueberries
- 2 tablespoons honey
- 1 tablespoon arrowroot powder
- 1 teaspoon vanilla extract
- 1/2 teaspoon ground cinnamon

PreparationTime: 15 minutes
Bake Time: 30 minutes
Total Time: 45 minutes
Serves: 6-8

Topping Ingredients:
- 1 cup rolled oats
- 1/2 cup almond flour
- 1/4 cup chopped walnuts
- 2 tablespoons coconut oil, melted
- 2 tablespoons honey
- 1/4 teaspoon sea salt

Instructions:

1. Preheat the oven to 375°F (190°C). Grease an 8x8-inch baking dish.

2. In a large bowl, gently toss together the diced pears, blueberries, honey, arrowroot powder, vanilla extract, and cinnamon until well combined.

3. In a separate bowl, mix together the rolled oats, almond flour, chopped walnuts, melted coconut oil, honey, and sea salt until the mixture resembles a crumbly topping.

4. Spread the pear and blueberry filling evenly into the prepared baking dish. Sprinkle the oat-walnut topping over the top.

5. Bake for 25-30 minutes, or until the topping is golden brown and the fruit is bubbling.

6. Allow the crisp to cool for at least 15 minutes before serving.

7. Serve the Pear and Blueberry Crisp warm, with a scoop of vanilla Greek yogurt or a drizzle of unsweetened almond milk, if desired.

This Pear and Blueberry Crisp is a delicious and nutritious dessert option for those following a menopause diet. The combination of juicy pears, antioxidant-rich blueberries, and a crunchy, fiber-rich topping makes this a satisfying and nourishing treat.

The almond flour, rolled oats, and walnuts provide healthy fats, fiber, and protein, while the honey adds natural sweetness without refined sugar.

107. Dark Chocolate Dipped Strawberries

Ingredients:

- 12 fresh strawberries, washed and patted dry
- 4 ounces dark chocolate
(at least 70% cacao), chopped
- 1 tablespoon coconut oil

PreparationTime: 15 minutes
Chilling Time: 30 minutes
Total Time: 45 minutes
Serves: 12 strawberries

Instructions:

1. Line a baking sheet or plate with parchment paper.

2. In a double boiler or a heatproof bowl set over a saucepan of simmering water, melt the chopped dark chocolate and coconut oil, stirring occasionally, until smooth and fully combined.

3. Carefully dip each strawberry into the melted chocolate, coating about three-quarters of the berry. Gently tap off any excess chocolate.

4. Place the chocolate-dipped strawberries on the prepared baking sheet or plate.

5. Refrigerate the strawberries for at least 30 minutes, or until the chocolate has set.

6. Serve the Dark Chocolate Dipped Strawberries chilled.

These Dark Chocolate Dipped Strawberries are a delicious and nutritious treat for a menopause diet. Strawberries are rich in antioxidants, fiber, and vitamin C, while dark chocolate provides a good source of flavonoids and healthy fats.

The coconut oil used in the chocolate coating adds additional healthy fats and helps the chocolate set up nicely. This recipe is easy to make and can be a satisfying way to enjoy a sweet treat without too much added sugar.

Store any leftover chocolate-dipped strawberries in an airtight container in the refrigerator for up to 3 days.

108. Peach and Raspberry Cobbler

Ingredients:

- 4 cups sliced fresh or frozen peaches
- 2 cups fresh or frozen raspberries
- 2 tablespoons honey
- 1 tablespoon arrowroot powder
- 1 teaspoon vanilla extract
- 1/4 teaspoon ground cinnamon

Topping Ingredients:
- 1 cup whole wheat flour
- 1/2 cup almond flour
- 1/4 cup rolled oats
- 2 tablespoons coconut oil, melted
- 2 tablespoons honey
- 1/4 teaspoon sea salt

Sweet and Healthy Desserts

PreparationTime: 20 minutes
Bake Time: 30 minutes
Total Time: 50 minutes
Serves: 6-8

Filling

Instructions:

1. Preheat the oven to 375°F (190°C). Grease an 8x8-inch baking dish.

2. In a large bowl, gently toss together the sliced peaches, raspberries, honey, arrowroot powder, vanilla extract, and cinnamon until well combined.

3. In a separate bowl, mix together the whole wheat flour, almond flour, rolled oats, melted coconut oil, honey, and sea salt until the mixture resembles a crumbly topping.

4. Spread the peach and raspberry filling evenly into the prepared baking dish. Sprinkle the oat-flour topping over the top.

5. Bake for 25-30 minutes, or until the topping is golden brown and the fruit is bubbling.

6. Allow the cobbler to cool for at least 15 minutes before serving.

7. Serve the Peach and Raspberry Cobbler warm, with a scoop of vanilla Greek yogurt or a drizzle of unsweetened almond milk, if desired.

This Peach and Raspberry Cobbler is a delicious and nutritious dessert option for those following a menopause diet. The combination of juicy peaches, tart raspberries, and a crunchy, fiber-rich topping makes this a satisfying and nourishing treat.

The whole wheat flour, almond flour, and rolled oats provide complex carbohydrates, fiber, and healthy fats, while the honey adds natural sweetness without refined sugar. The cinnamon may also help to regulate blood sugar levels.

109. Protein-Packed Peanut Butter Cookies

Ingredients:

- 1 cup natural peanut butter (no added sugar)
- 1/2 cup unsweetened applesauce
- 1/4 cup honey
- 1 egg
- 1 scoop (about 30g) vanilla protein powder
- 1/4 cup ground flaxseed
- 1/2 teaspoon baking soda
- 1/4 teaspoon sea salt

PreparationTime: 10 minutes
Bake Time: 12 minutes
Total Time: 22 minutes
Yields: 12 cookies

Instructions:

1. Preheat the oven to 350°F (175°C). Line a baking sheet with parchment paper.

2. In a medium bowl, combine the peanut butter, unsweetened applesauce, honey, and egg. Mix until well blended.

3. Add the vanilla protein powder, ground flaxseed, baking soda, and sea salt to the wet ingredients. Stir until a thick, cookie dough-like consistency forms.

4. Scoop the dough by the tablespoonful and place the cookies about 2 inches apart on the prepared baking sheet.

5. Bake for 10-12 minutes, or until the cookies are lightly golden around the edges.

6. Allow the cookies to cool on the baking sheet for 5 minutes before transferring them to a wire rack to cool completely.

These Protein-Packed Peanut Butter Cookies are a delicious and nutritious treat for a menopause diet. The peanut butter provides a good source of protein, healthy fats, and fiber, while the protein powder, flaxseed, and applesauce add additional nutrients.

The honey is used as a natural sweetener, and the baking soda helps to create a soft, chewy texture. These cookies are a great option for a post-workout snack, a satisfying dessert, or a quick energy boost.

Store the cookies in an airtight container at room temperature for up to 5 days.

110. Coconut Yogurt with Pineapple and Granola

Ingredients:

- 2 cups unsweetened coconut yogurt
- 1 cup diced fresh pineapple
- 1/2 cup homemade granola (see recipe below)
- 2 tablespoons unsweetened shredded coconut

Homemade Granola Ingredients:
- 2 cups rolled oats
- 1/2 cup chopped walnuts
- 1/4 cup unsweetened shredded coconut
- 2 tablespoons coconut oil, melted
- 2 tablespoons honey
- 1/2 teaspoon ground cinnamon
- 1/4 teaspoon sea salt

Sweet and Healthy Desserts

PreparationTime: 10 minutes
Total Time: 10 minutes
Serves: 4

Instructions:
Homemade Granola:
1. Preheat the oven to 325°F (165°C). Line a baking sheet with parchment paper.
2. In a large bowl, combine the rolled oats, chopped walnuts, and unsweetened shredded coconut.
3. Drizzle the melted coconut oil and honey over the oat mixture, and sprinkle with cinnamon and sea salt. Stir until well coated.
4. Spread the granola mixture evenly on the prepared baking sheet.
5. Bake for 15-20 minutes, stirring halfway, until lightly golden. Allow to cool completely.

Coconut Yogurt with Pineapple and Granola:
1. Divide the coconut yogurt evenly among 4 serving bowls or glasses.
2. Top each serving with 1/4 cup of diced fresh pineapple, 2 tablespoons of the homemade granola, and 1/2 tablespoon of unsweetened shredded coconut.
3. Serve immediately and enjoy!

This Coconut Yogurt with Pineapple and Granola is a delicious and nutritious breakfast or snack option for a menopause diet. The coconut yogurt provides a good source of probiotics, while the pineapple and granola add fiber, healthy fats, and natural sweetness.

The homemade granola is made with wholesome ingredients like rolled oats, walnuts, and coconut, making it a nutritious and satisfying topping. This dish is easy to prepare and can be customized with your favorite fruits or nuts.

Creating Balanced Menus

Meal planning is an essential part of maintaining a healthy diet, especially during menopause. Planning your meals ahead of time ensures that you have nutritious options readily available, reduces stress, and helps you stay on track with your dietary goals.

Steps to Create Balanced Menus
- Assess Your Nutritional Needs: Consider your specific dietary requirements, such as the need for calcium, vitamin D, phytoestrogens, and omega-3 fatty acids.

- Plan for Variety: Include a mix of proteins, carbohydrates, healthy fats, and plenty of fruits and vegetables in your meals.

- Balance Macronutrients: Ensure that each meal includes a balance of macronutrients—protein, fats, and carbohydrates—to keep you satiated and energized.

- Incorporate Snacks: Plan for healthy snacks to keep your energy levels stable throughout the day.

- Stay Hydrated: Include beverages like water, herbal teas, and nutrient-rich smoothies in your plan.

Sample Weekly Menu
Monday:
- Breakfast: Greek yogurt with berries and flaxseeds
- Lunch: Quinoa salad with chickpeas, cucumber, and feta
- Dinner: Baked salmon with steamed broccoli and sweet potatoes
- Snack: Apple slices with almond butter

Tuesday:
- Breakfast: Overnight oats with chia seeds and fresh fruit
- Lunch: Lentil soup with a side of mixed greens
- Dinner: Grilled chicken with quinoa and roasted vegetables
- Snack: Carrot sticks with hummus

Wednesday:
- Breakfast: Smoothie with spinach, banana, and almond milk
- Lunch: Turkey and avocado wrap with whole-grain tortilla
- Dinner: Stir-fried tofu with vegetables and brown rice
- Snack: Handful of walnuts

Thursday:
- Breakfast: Scrambled eggs with spinach and whole-grain toast
- Lunch: Tuna salad with mixed greens and olive oil dressing
- Dinner: Spaghetti squash with marinara sauce and ground turkey
- Snack: Greek yogurt with honey

Friday:
- Breakfast: Cottage cheese with pineapple and chia seeds
- Lunch: Chickpea and vegetable stir-fry
- Dinner: Grilled shrimp with quinoa and asparagus
- Snack: Sliced bell peppers with guacamole

Saturday:
- Breakfast: Avocado toast with a poached egg
- Lunch: Black bean soup with a side of whole-grain bread
- Dinner: Baked cod with roasted Brussels sprouts and brown rice
- Snack: Smoothie with berries and protein powder

Sunday:
- Breakfast: Oatmeal with almonds and fresh fruit
- Lunch: Greek salad with grilled chicken
- Dinner: Vegetable and tofu kebabs with couscous
- Snack: Fresh fruit salad

Shopping Lists and Pantry Essentials

Having a well-stocked pantry makes meal preparation easier and ensures you have healthy options available at all times.

Pantry Essentials

- Whole Grains: Quinoa, brown rice, oats, whole-grain pasta

- Legumes: Lentils, chickpeas, black beans

- Nuts and Seeds: Almonds, walnuts, chia seeds, flaxseeds

- Healthy Oils: Olive oil, avocado oil, coconut oil

- Spices and Herbs: Turmeric, ginger, garlic, basil, parsley

- Condiments: Soy sauce, balsamic vinegar, Dijon mustard

- Canned Goods: Tomatoes, tuna, salmon, coconut milk

- Baking Essentials: Whole-wheat flour, almond flour, baking powder

Fresh Produce

- Fruits: Berries, apples, bananas, oranges

- Vegetables: Spinach, kale, broccoli, bell peppers, carrots

- Proteins: Chicken breast, salmon, tofu, eggs

- Dairy/Alternatives: Greek yogurt, almond milk, cheese

Tips for Efficient Meal Prep

Meal prep can save time and ensure you have healthy meals ready to go, reducing the temptation to opt for less nutritious options.

Meal Prep Strategies

- Plan Your Menu: Start with a weekly menu plan and create a shopping list based on the recipes you'll be preparing.

- Batch Cooking: Cook large batches of grains, proteins, and vegetables that can be used in various meals throughout the week.

- Portioning: Divide meals into individual portions to make it easy to grab and go.

- Storage: Use airtight containers to keep food fresh. Label them with the date to keep track of freshness.

- Pre-Cut Ingredients: Chop vegetables and fruits in advance to save time during the week.

Sample Meal Prep Routine

Sunday:
- Cook a batch of quinoa and brown rice.
- Roast a tray of mixed vegetables.
- Grill chicken breasts and bake salmon fillets.
- Prepare a large salad to be used throughout the week.
- Make a batch of overnight oats for the first few days.

Portion Control and Storage

Understanding portion sizes and proper storage techniques can help you maintain a balanced diet and reduce food waste.

Portion Control Tips

- Use Smaller Plates: This can help control portion sizes and prevent overeating.
- Measure Servings: Use measuring cups or a food scale to ensure accurate portion sizes.
- Balanced Plates: Aim for a plate that's half vegetables, a quarter protein, and a quarter whole grains.

Storage Tips

- Refrigeration: Store perishable items in the fridge and consume them within a few days.
- Freezing: Freeze portions of cooked grains, proteins, and soups for longer storage.
- Labeling: Label containers with the date of preparation to keep track of freshness.

By incorporating these meal planning and preparation strategies into your routine, you can ensure that you have nutritious and delicious meals ready to support your health and well-being during menopause. Meal planning not only saves time and reduces stress but also helps you stay committed to a balanced and healthful diet.